HOMEOPATHY IN AMERICA

HOMEOPATHY
IN
AMERICA
THE RISE AND FALL
OF A MEDICAL HERESY

MARTIN KAUFMAN

THE JOHNS HOPKINS PRESS
BALTIMORE AND LONDON

The Johns Hopkins Press, Baltimore, Maryland 21218
The Johns Hopkins Press Ltd., London

Library of Congress Catalog Card Number 79-149741

International Standard Book Number 0-8018-1238-0

To my parents,
Irving and Rose Kaufman

CONTENTS

PREFACE

WHILE READING a number of old medical journals in search of a likely dissertation topic, I became curious about the bitter and often sarcastic comments about the homeopathic practitioners. Indeed, the orthodox physicians seemed to make sport by attacking their unorthodox colleagues. As I delved deeper into the sources, the story became more and more interesting. The result of my enthusiasm is this study of the relationship between the orthodox profession and the homeopaths, covering the period from 1820 to 1960. While writing, it became necessary to trace the history of homeopathy until well into the twentieth century, in order to make the changing relationship more intelligible and to provide continuity.

The history of homeopathy is interesting as history and can prove valuable for a number of reasons. The medical profession has always been faced by the competition from heretical sects. Based upon varying theories, practicing differing methods, all the sects claimed to provide more effective and safer treatment than could the allopaths, as the orthodox practitioners were called. The homeopaths were only one of a long line of unconventional physicians, yet the history of homeopathy is to a large extent the history of every unorthodox sect. They all have encountered the same reaction from the regular profession and seem to have undergone similar metamorphoses. Indeed, in the history of osteopathy one can easily recognize the road previously traveled by the homeopaths. Perhaps present and future medical sectarians can learn from the history of homeopathy, and so can be better prepared to face the changing medical world. Similarly, the orthodox profession may be able to learn how to handle future sectarians.

In any case, in the course of my research and writing I have become indebted to various organizations and individuals. Part of the research was financed by the Josiah Macy, Jr. Foundation, and I would like to thank Dr. John Z. Bowers and the Macy Foundation for their generous assistance. Professor John Duffy of Tulane University is deserving of more credit than can possibly be expressed, since he developed my interest in medical history and guided this study from its inception. I am also obliged to Professors William R. Hogan, also of Tulane, and Charles G. Roland of the University of Kentucky. The staff members of a number of libraries were especially helpful, including Richard Wolfe of the rare book division of Harvard University's Francis Countway Library, Archie Motley of the Chicago Historical Society, Dr. Robert Warner and Mrs. Janice Earle of the Michigan Historical Collections, and Manfred Wasserman and Dorothy Hanks of the National Library of Medicine, at Bethesda, Maryland. References to the William Prescott and John W. Francis Papers are made with permission of the Manuscript Division, The New York Public Library, Astor, Lenox and Tilden Foundations.

Kay Vargo and James Lavelle of the American Foundation for Homeopathy were exceedingly helpful in offering me free access to their manuscript collection. Dr. Robert Buck and Dr. F. Thomas Gephart of the Massachusetts Medical Society were also helpful in allowing me to see the records of the early boards of trial. Warren Albert and Oliver Field of the American Medical Association were of assistance, although the A.M.A. has very few records from before the 1920's.

I am deeply indebted to my friend and colleague Dr. Charles A. Watson of Roger Williams College, who has read and criticized the entire manuscript. Dr. Leslie Hanawalt, an expert on the medical history of Michigan, kindly consented to read the chapter on the Ann Arbor "embroglio," and his many suggestions were helpful. Most of the newspapers cited were found in the newspaper division of the Boston Public Library, where James Monahan devoted many hours to locating the various journals. Most of the typing was done by Angela Musto. Finally, for her assistance and constant encouragement, my wife Henrietta has my everlasting appreciation.

HOMEOPATHY IN AMERICA

I

THE AGE OF HEROIC MEDICINE

THE PERIOD from the 1780's to the 1850's has often been called the age of heroic medicine. For most ailments, physicians prescribed extensive blood-letting. In addition, they administered huge doses of calomel and other dangerous mineral drugs, as well as purgatives and emetics to cleanse the system of all irritants. Venesection was an age-old remedy, but by the turn of the century virtually every disease was treated by bleeding.[1]

Through his writings and his teachings at the University of Edinburgh, William Cullen provided much of the theoretical basis for the increase in the practice of blood-letting. Like a number of his colleagues, he devised a system of medical practice based upon his observations of fevers. He identified the stages of fever as a preliminary cold state followed by a hot one, which in turn lead to general debility. Cullen thought that there must be some relationship between that sequence and a "spasm of the extreme vessels," a physiological change he had observed in fevers of every type. According to his theory, the spasm irritated the heart and arteries, and it continued to upset the system until the spasm was overcome.[2] Treatment could not be too severe, as fever in itself was debilitating. The spasm, Cullen said, could be eliminated by means of an anti-phlogistic regimen, which consisted of moderate blood-letting, purging, applications of cold

[1] Benjamin Rush, *Medical Inquiries and Observations* (3d ed.; Philadelphia, 1809), IV, 396, 411. See also Joseph I. Waring, "The Influence of Benjamin Rush on the Practice of Bleeding in South Carolina," *Bulletin of the History of Medicine* 35 (May–June 1961): 230–37.

[2] William Cullen, *First Lines of the Practice of Physic* (New York, 1801), I, 37, 40, 70–72. For a thorough examination of Cullen's medical thought, see Lester S. King, *The Medical World of the Eighteenth Century* (Chicago, 1958), pp. 139ff.

water, and attention to the diet and comfort of the patient. Although himself a moderate in the use of this practice, Cullen provided much of the rationale for its subsequent increase.

Benjamin Rush, one of Cullen's students, carried the theory to an extreme with his doctrine of the "unity of fevers." He accepted his teacher's idea that the spasm of the extreme vessels provided the morbid excitement in fever, but, unlike Cullen, he ascribed all disease to "capillary tension." While Cullen produced massive lists of diseases, each with different symptoms and treatments, Rush asserted that there was only one disease, and thus only one cure. That cure was blood-letting, purging, and more blood-letting. He had such confidence in the lancet that he was willing to remove up to four-fifths of the blood in the body if necessary to alleviate the symptoms.[3] According to the Rushian system, the irritation was to be removed through bleeding and purging; recuperation was to be speeded through the use of tonics and careful diet controls. If purging failed to suppress the fever, the resort was to venesection.[4]

In his lectures on the practice of medicine, Rush demonstrated his faith in extensive blood-letting. He began his 1798 class at the medical department of the University of Pennsylvania with the comment that he rejected Cullen's as well as every other system of medical practice. His own system, he asserted, was far superior to any other. Rush graphically described the difference between his system and that of Cullen: "We will suppose the Doctor to have a house containing 100 rooms, each having a different Lock; of course he must have an equal number of different Keys to open them— now I am capable of entering every apartment of my House with the assistance of a Single Key."[5] That key was massive blood-letting. Urging his students never to stop the flow of blood once it was started, Rush said that bleeding "but once or twice . . . is like untying a Tyger & not destroying him afterwards." "Tis a very hard Matter to bleed a Patient to Death," he assured his students, "provided the Blood be not drawn from a Vital Part." Rush noted that he had been ridiculed by his colleagues for bleeding his patients "till they were as pale as Jersey Veal." Not a man to wilt under attack, the Philadelphia physician defended his use of the lancet with an

[3] See Rush, *Medical Inquiries and Observations,* IV, 348–53.

[4] For an examination of Rush's theories, see Nathan Goodman, *Benjamin Rush: Physician and Citizen* (Philadelphia, 1934), pp. 229–54, and King, *Medical World of the Eighteenth Century,* pp. 147ff.

[5] Alexander Clendinen, comp., "Notes on the practice of Physic, from the Lectures of Benjamin Rush, at the University of Pennsylvania, 1798," pp. 1–2; MS in Joseph Toner Collection, Library of Congress.

inspiring lecture. "I would sooner die with my Lancet in my hand," he said, "than give it up while I had Breath to maintain it or a hand to use it."[6]

The ensuing lectures of that term were devoted to a survey of the various diseases, descriptions of their symptoms, and methods of cure. The treatments almost exclusively consisted of blood-letting, even to the extent of one to two hundred ounces. In his final lecture, Rush urged his students to "do homage to the Lancet . . .. I say venerate the Lancet Gentlemen."[7] Medical educators of the first half of the nineteenth century continued to advocate massive blood-letting as a cure for a variety of ailments, although there were always some physicians who doubted the efficacy of such harsh therapeutics.

In general, the heroic practice consisted of bleeding, cupping, blistering, purging, and sweating.[8] Blood-letting was intended to moderate vascular excitement, reduce inflammation, relieve congestion, alleviate spasm and pain, relax muscles, and arrest hemorrhage. General blood-letting was done by venesection, the opening of a vein and the release of several ounces to several pounds of blood, depending upon the ailment and the courage of the physician. Local blood-letting was practiced by means of leeches, cupping and scarificating. Cupping, according to one textbook, was effected when the "removal of atmospheral pressure, by application of glasses partially exhausted of air, produces a determination of blood to the capillaries of a part, and it is afterwards readily drawn by scarification."[9]

Leeches were used in external inflammations, in situations where cups were inconvenient or inaccessible, and on infants, who were not considered strong enough to undergo cupping. In 1858 Frederick Stearns, an editor of the *Peninsular and Independent Medical Journal*, published an article intended to instruct the reader in the fine art of leeching. Leeches had not found their way into the western world in large quantities, due to the high cost of transportation and the problem of spoilage. Fortunately for medical science, and unfortunately for the patient, the improved forms of transit

---

[6] Ibid., pp. 11–16.

[7] Ibid., pp. 64–67. Rush venerated the lancet to such an extent that he thought it most important to bleed infants and children, who were difficult to depress in other ways. See his *Medical Inquiries and Observations*, IV, 300.

[8] The following discussion of heroic practices is derived from several texts, especially John B. Biddle, *Materia Medica for the Use of Students* (8th ed.; Philadelphia, 1878) and John B. Beck, *Lectures on Materia Medica and Therapeutics* (New York, 1856).

[9] Biddle, *Materia Medica*, pp. 18–19.

brought about a price reduction in the late 1850's. Stearns felt it necessary to describe the methods of leeching, so that the western physician could benefit from his knowledge. "Having determined upon the number to be used," the doctor should "place them in a cupping glass, over the part affected." It might be necessary, he continued, to "partly fill the cupping-glass with water, as they will bite more readily when covered by it. When they have attached themselves, the cup can be gently removed, and the part surrounded by a soft cloth, which will absorb the moisture and blood, and catch the Leeches when they drop off." "If a flow of blood greater than that swallowed by the Leech is desired, it must be excited after the leech drops off, by warm fomentations or poultices." [10] Presumably, once having read this article, the western physician could use his newly learned therapeutic to benefit humanity, especially the infants who were too frail to be cupped.

In the practice of blistering, a harsh substance was placed or burned upon the skin, causing a second degree burn. Since it nearly always became infected, the wound would suppurate. The pus was usually taken as evidence that the infection was being drawn out of the system. The customary blister consisted of local irritants, such as Spanish fly, cantharides, or tartar emetic.

Purging was effected in various ways. Emetics were employed to induce vomiting, and cathartics were used to evacuate waste from the bowels. Emetics were intended to cleanse the stomach, expel foreign bodies, or to depress the vascular and muscular systems. The leading emetics were ipecac, tartar emetic, and sulphate of zinc. Cathartics served much the same purposes as emetics, and the leading laxatives were tamarind, manna, cassia, castor oil, magnesia, rhubarb, and senna. The more drastic cathartics were jalap, croton oil, and calomel.[11] Sweating, another heroic practice, was produced by diaphoretics (substances which promote secretions through the skin). Most emetics, especially antimony and ipecac, were well able to produce sweating. It could also be produced by altering external conditions, such as heating the rooms, wrapping the patient in warm clothing, and so forth.[12]

These were the five mainstays of heroic practice, along with large doses of calomel (mercurous chloride). Calomel was noted for its effect upon the salivary glands, as it increased secretion to great extent. According to

---

[10] *Peninsular and Independent Medical Journal* I (July 1858): 220–23.
[11] See Biddle, *Materia Medica*, pp. 247–53, 253–84; Beck, *Lectures on Materia Medica*, pp. 50ff., 90ff.
[12] Biddle, *Materia Medica*, p. 285; Beck, *Lectures on Materia Medica*, pp. 191–206.

Professor John B. Beck of the College of Physicians and Surgeons of the University of the State of New York, it was often given "without regard to anything but the quantity that can be given." Although he recognized the dangers involved in the administration of calomel, Beck recommended it in fevers, inflammations, tonsilitis, bronchitis, dysentery, after venesection in pleurisy and pneumonia, hepatitis, and to promote secretions of blood and other fluids. In laryngitis he prescribed calomel "carried to salivation," and "in as large doses as the system will bear." The net results of such massive doses were salivation, loosening of the teeth, falling of the hair, and other symptoms of acute mercuric poisoning.[13]

Medical students from the 1790's until the 1860's and 1870's were taught that massive blood-letting was the standard cure for nearly all ailments. As the nineteenth century advanced, however, many leading physicians raised their voices in opposition to these drastic treatments. In 1835 Jacob Bigelow read a paper "On Self-Limited Diseases," which has been called the first effective protest against heroic medicine in the United States.[14] This was followed in 1840 by the comments of Dr. Samuel Jackson, who said that the "least important part of the science . . . is the dosing of patients with medicine."[15] Jackson questioned the value of the medication used by so many of the doctors, at the same time that Bigelow and others were calling for a return to the healing powers of nature in the treatment of the ill.[16]

A survey of medical textbooks indicates that blood-letting and the antiphlogistic regimen continued to be recommended during the entire antebellum period, even in the face of such determined opposition. James Thacher, in his 1826 *American Modern Practice*, emphasized the use of emetics, cold water compresses, and rest. He added, however, that blood-letting was the most direct means of diminishing the quantity of fluid in the system. He did recognize that it was not the panacea that Rush had asserted it to be. Thacher noted, for example, that it caused debility and was hazardous to patients suffering from the fevers which were particularly

[13] Beck, *Lectures on Materia Medica*, pp. 161–90.

[14] Jacob Bigelow, *Nature in Disease* (Boston, 1854), pp. 1–58. See also Richard H. Shryock, *Medicine and Society in America: 1660–1860* (New York, 1960), pp. 131–32.

[15] Address to Medical Graduates, University of Pennsylvania, 1840, cited in Shryock, *Medicine and Society*, p. 131. See also Charles S. Bryan, "Bloodletting in American Medicine, 1830–1892," *Bulletin of the History of Medicine* 38 (November–December 1964): 520.

[16] For the opposition to heroic medicine in one state, see John Duffy, *Rudolph Matas History of Medicine in Louisiana* (Baton Rouge, 1962), II, 5–6.

debilitating in themselves, such as typhus. Despite his caution about general blood-letting, Thacher insisted that even the most conservative physician would admit that "local blood-letting by means of leeches or cupping" was beneficial in certain conditions, especially when there was "much head-ach, or dilerium [sic], accompanied by flushing of the countenance and redness of the eyes." He added that in those cases, "the application of a few leeches to the temples, or the scarificator and cupping-glasses to the same part, or to the nape of the neck, has often diminished the symptoms; sometimes carried them off entirely, and arrested the progress of the fever." [17]

Thacher prescribed sweating and purging to reduce vascular tension. He claimed that blisters were "decidedly beneficial" in relieving local pains and congestion and that "every practitioner has experienced their utility, when the brain, stomach, lungs, &c., have been affected." [18] Calomel, he said, had been used for the past fifty years, especially in New England. Combined with either jalap or rhubarb, it had proven to be an excellent purgative. Thacher recommended one to three grains of calomel every four to six hours, until "its effects on the system become evident, by a moderate ptya-lism [salivation]." In order to prevent stomach and bowel irritation by the calomel acting alone, Thacher suggested the combination of calomel and opium. [19]

In 1833, in the second edition of William P. Dewees's textbook on the *Practice of Physic*, the author noted that bleeding was so universally ac-cepted that it had "almost become a domestic remedy." [20] Twelve years later John Eberle wrote in his widely read text that bloodletting was the best means to moderate "febrile excitement." [21] In 1849 George B. Wood con-tinued in much the same vein, but warned that bleeding to syncope (i.e., unconsciousness) was injurious, while at the same time recommending local bleeding by leeching or cupping. [22]

Throughout his education, then, the medical student was taught the bene-fits derived from heroic practice. Doctors' daybooks, journals, and diaries and letters of the patients indicate that this knowledge was put to very good use in daily practice. Dr. Moses G. Elmer, for example, of New

[17] James Thacher, *American Modern Practice* (Boston, 1826), pp. 201–16.
[18] Ibid., pp. 210–11.
[19] Ibid., pp. 212–14.
[20] William P. Dewees, *A Practice of Physic* (2d ed.; Philadelphia, 1833), p. 75.
[21] John Eberle, *A Treatise on the Practice of Medicine* (Philadelphia, 1845), I, 113–14.
[22] George B. Wood, *A Treatise on the Practice of Medicine* (2d ed.; Philadel-phia, 1849), I, 199–202.

Providence, New Jersey, over a three-month period in 1786 administered to one patient sal ammoniac, cream of tartar, an antimonial mixture, emetic and anodyne pills, boluses (large pill masses), and various other powders. In addition, he let blood at least fourteen times, and blistered the patient's head and shoulders twenty-four times. To demonstrate the lasting power of Homus Americanus, the patient "apparently lived to pay a bill of over 39 pounds."[23]

William Maclay, the United States Senator from Pennsylvania, recorded in his journal the details of his illness and treatment in 1789. Suffering from rheumatism in his hip and leg, he summoned a physician. Two doctors arrived, and despite Maclay's complaint that the pain was centered in his knee, they urged that the good Senator undergo a full course of antimonials to cleanse his stomach. Maclay's journal demonstrates his anger at the quality of medical care. On September 8 he recorded that the doctors did "not call to-day, and it seems like delivering me from half of my misery."[24] Even Dr. Philip Syng Physick, perhaps the leading American surgeon of his day, in 1807 prescribed leeches and general bleeding for a bad case of inflamed eyes. Benjamin Rush noted that Physick had discovered, correctly, that bleeding was even beneficial in the case of dislocations. The blood loss and resultant unconsciousness relaxed his patients and made manipulation easier for the doctor.[25]

Even George Washington, who received the best medical care of the day, spent his last hours undergoing heroic treatment. On December 14, 1799, the former President came down with a severe sore throat. It was inflamed and gave him some difficulty in breathing. His overseer removed a pint of blood, but it provided no relief. A physician was called, who soon after his arrival applied a blister to the throat and let another pint of blood. At three o'clock that afternoon, two other doctors came to consult with the first one, and by a vote of two to one they decided to let more blood, removing a quart that time. They reported that the blood flowed "slow and thick." By then the President was dehydrated, and it would seem that the doctors must have had to squeeze out the final drops of blood. Washington died sometime between ten and eleven that same night. In his case heroic

---

[23] David Cowen, *Medicine and Health in New Jersey: A History* (Princeton, 1964), p. 19.

[24] *Journal of William Maclay,* edited by Edgar S. Maclay (New York, 1890), pp. 149–50.

[25] George Clymer to Samuel Meredith [Philadelphia], April 2, 1807, MS in Dreer Collection, Historical Society of Pennsylvania, Philadelphia; Rush, *Medical Inquiries and Observations,* IV, 378–79.

treatment consisted of the removal of at least four pints of blood, blistering, and a dose of calomel. Perhaps he would have died in any case, but the treatment certainly provided no relief.[26]

The diary of Reverend John Monteith of Detroit is a gold mine of information on medicine and public health in the west. Through its entries, one can see the entire course of heroic medicine. In 1820 his wife became ill during a visit to Ohio. On September 19 Monteith recorded in his diary that she was "taking calomel." Two days later: "Dr. Wright applies some plasters, continuing calomel. Feet bathed in warm water." The following day he wrote that "salivation begins," which, as noted earlier, was the first sign of acute mercurial poisoning. On September 25 the physician discontinued the calomel, and the next day the patient is reported to have taken a dose of sulphur, possibly as a cathartic. Three days later she was given magnesia and "calomel cathartick." On October 2, Mrs. Monteith was instructed to take pills to keep her bowels open, along with doses of tea of valerian and castor oil to provide nourishment and a gentle stimulant. Two days later Dr. Wright applied several blisters and prescribed drinks of camphor and water. On October 5 the patient was "Given up by all three doctors," but the following day the good Reverend recorded in his diary that the "Blisters have drawn well, especially those on [the] head. Her hair is shaved." She finally died on October 9, after having suffered through almost every aspect of heroic medicine.[27]

Dr. William Prescott of Concord, New Hampshire, wrote a number of his colleagues in 1827 to determine what they were prescribing for acute enteritis. Dr. R. D. Mussey replied: "I bleed largely and repeatedly, and give opium & calomel (if the stomach will bear) [;] if not opium alone in Such doses & at such intervals as will keep down the pain." He continued: "When a cathartick is judged necessary I give two parts of castor oil & one of spirit of turpentine, enough to move the bowels three or four times." In more severe cases, Mussey applied a large blister.[28] A second physician, Dr. A. Twitchell, responded by stating that he began "by bleeding *ad dilgerium* or till a very sensible impression is made upon the system." When he bled, he asserted: "I always find that one taking 20 or 30

[26] *American Heritage* 6 (August 1955): 43ff.

[27] John Monteith Diaries, 1808–1821, 2 vols., photostats in Burton Historical Collection, Detroit Public Library, cited in Fannie Anderson, *Doctors Under Three Flags* (Detroit, 1951), pp. 138–40.

[28] Mussey to Prescott, June 27, 1827, MS in William Prescott Papers, New York Public Library.

ounces at once & suddenly has more effect than twice that quantity taken at several times." "After making a suitable impression upon the inflammation by the lancet," Twitchell usually applied "a large blister over the abdomen—& administer 20 or 30 grains of calomel with 2 grs. of extract of Hyosicanda or Belladonna." The dose was repeated once or twice over a twenty-four hour period, "until purging is produced." If that failed to evacuate the patient, he would "give an injection of a decoction of tobacco of the strength of 20 or 30 grs. to half a pint & repeat till some effect is perceived." [29]

Dr. Matthias Spalding, in his response to Prescott's letter, wrote that he did not bleed "as freely as many do in this disease, or [as] indiscriminately." He relied chiefly upon mild cathartics, such as neutral salts, senna, manna, and castor oil, and he reported that this was more effective than "copious & frequent bleedings." He did resort to "a large blister," as well as to injections of opium or a combination of opium and calomel in practically every case.[30]

The closer to the frontier, the more heroic were the doses. Advances in medical science were slow to reach the scattered settlements of the west and the south. Dr. John P. Harrison read a paper before the Hamilton County Medical Club, of Cincinnati, on July 3, 1845, which illustrates the exceptional courage of the frontier physician. He recommended "herculian doses of Calomel & opium." One of the commentators at the meeting noted that "None but a Kentuckyan would give or take such doses." The commentator suggested that Harrison might do well to mention "the antidotes for an overdose." [31] The following July, Harrison spoke about his trip to Mississippi. He told his colleagues that calomel was "rarely given at the South in doses of more than 15 to 20 gn." The large doses recommended by "Prof. Cook of Transylvania, formerly so much in vogue" he reported to be "almost entirely abandoned." Harrison concluded by noting that quinine had superseded the use of calomel in fevers and that cupping was very popular in the treatment of "congestive diseases." [32]

Harrison's reference was to Dr. John E. Cooke, who encouraged the administration of massive doses of purgatives. According to Cooke's own theory, disease weakened heart action and produced an accumulation of

[29] Twitchell to Prescott, Keene, New Hampshire, June 28, 1827, in ibid.
[30] Spalding to Prescott, Amherst, New Hampshire, June 29, 1827, in ibid.
[31] Hamilton County Medical Club, Minutes, 1842–1850, MS in National Library of Medicine, Bethesda, Maryland.
[32] Ibid., July 8, 1846.

blood in the larger veins. As a remedy for virtually every ailment, Professor Cooke prescribed large doses of calomel. He announced that if "calomel did not salivate, and opium did not constipate, there is no telling what we could do in the practice of physic." It is also said that he administered thirteen tablespoons of calomel to one patient during a three-day bout with cholera. Needless to say, the patient survived neither the disease nor the treatment.[33]

The changes in medical care can easily be traced in the state of Louisiana. During the first three decades of the nineteenth century, the lancet and calomel provided the major weapons of the medical profession in the struggle with disease. Reverend Theodore Clapp, a prominent New Orleans minister, wrote in 1856 that in an earlier epidemic he had seen a physician on "his first visit to a patient, who had been ill but four hours, take from him, by the lancet, fifty ounces of blood at one time." The patient lost consciousness, was revived, and the doctor then "ordered him to swallow, at once, three hundred grains of calomel and gamboge."[34] In 1833 a reviewer in the *Western Journal of Medical and Physical Sciences* said that the "practice of our brethren of the lower Mississippi, is well known to be characterized by great boldness and energy. The lancet and calomel, particularly the last, constitute their anchor of hope, in the endemic fevers of that region."[35]

In 1844, however, the editor of the *New Orleans Medical Journal* noted that there had been a change in medical practice during the past ten years. The Southern physician had reportedly become "more moderate" in his use of emetics and cathartics, and rather than relying upon harsh purgatives to treat fever, he used mild evacuants, venesection, cupping, leeching, and cold applications. "Quinine, instead of calomel," the editor noted, "is now considered in the South, the *Sampson* of the *Materia Medica*."[36] Twelve years later, in 1856, Dr. M. Morton Dowler spoke of even greater changes. He reported that the treatment of "acute and febrile diseases" by "bloodletting, purgation, mercurialization, starvation, and other depressing, debilitating, and depletory measures, usually denominated antiphlogistic" had given way to more modern therapeutics.[37]

---

[33] Howard A. Kelly, *Cyclopedia of American Medical Biography* (Philadelphia and London, 1912), I, 199–201.

[34] Duffy, *Matas History*, II, 5.

[35] 7 (1833–34): 187, cited in ibid., II, 5.

[36] 1 (1844): 247–48, cited in ibid., II, 6.

[37] Dowler, "Remarks on Therapeutics," *New Orleans Medical and Surgical Journal* 12 (1855–56): 49, cited in ibid., II, 7.

In the 1830's, according to Southern medical writers, synopal bleeding was introduced on a large scale at the same time as was quinine. These two remedies replaced calomel as the mainstay of the profession. Yet while medical writers devoted time and energy to their theoretical debates, the average physician continued to purge, bleed, blister, and administer calomel and opium. By examination of the records of drug houses and pharmacists, Professor John Duffy demonstrated that there was very little change in medication from the 1820's to the 1850's. Medicine most frequently sold included paregoric, "blue pills" (mercury), castor oil, salts of tartar, Epsom salts, and so forth. Spring and thumb lancets for bleeding were always in constant demand, and in the 1850's an order sent to one plantation included a spring lancet, two thumb lancets, six dozen cups, and one scarificator.[38]

Medical care left much to be desired during the age of heroic medicine, but it should be recognized that the average patient insisted upon receiving the treatment which was currently most popular. Physicians of every age have found that the most recent medical miracle was always in demand for every and any ailment. If not purged, bled, and sweated, it can be expected that the early-nineteenth-century patient would have had little respect for his physician. Whether the cure-all was blood-letting, alcohol, opium, stimulants, or the penicillin and sulfa drugs of the twentieth century, patients have insisted upon it. Woe to the doctor who is unwilling to accede to the demands of his patients.

Senator William Woodbridge demonstrated this in a letter to his wife in 1842. He described the various methods used to combat the violent influenza which had attacked the nation's capital. These included "bleeding,— but cupping far more generally—blisters—mustard poultices—& sudorifics [which induce sweating]," "accompanied of course by cathartics." He proceeded to give his wife some advice: "if at any time you should need *bleeding*—you will find (if *our* physicians have the proper treatment & understand) that the use of the *cupping* glasses will, with you—be found the most sure & convenient." Cupping was then considered a cure-all, and patients frequently insisted on that mode of treatment.[39]

John P. Brashears, of Livingston Parish, Louisiana, writing his autobiography in the 1890's, demonstrated that the general faith of the public in calomel almost matched that of the physician. He wrote: "They used

38 Duffy, *Matas History*, II, 10–12, 20, 28–29.
39 William Woodbridge to his wife, Washington, D.C., January 12, 1842, MS in Woodbridge Papers, Burton Historical Collection, Detroit Public Library.

blue mast a good deal for people who had liver complaints, and it was a wonderful medicine, so the doctors said, but calamine [calomel] was the principal medicine. Those days there was so much malaria through the country, till you couldn't hardly live without calamine [calomel]."[40] Professor Duffy has noted of calomel that "any country physician who failed to prescribe it would undoubtedly have aroused suspicion as to his qualifications in the minds of his patients."[41]

Certainly a majority of patients had confidence in heroic medical practice, but there were many who had their doubts, doubts which were reinforced by the openly proclaimed skepticism and the unwillingness of the more forward-looking physicians to prescribe bleeding, blistering, and the anti-phlogistic regimen. The increasing opposition to heroic practice within the medical profession led to a corresponding increase in popular distrust of the physician. This can be seen from a number of private letters, as well as through newspapers and magazines.

Charles M. Bull, of Detroit, for instance, in 1832 wrote to his father of the treatment given him for an attack of cholera: "I was in the first place bled 3 times & Physicked almost to deth." In a subsequent letter he noted that "the Doctors have got an idea into their heads that they must give calomel for evry complaint [;] they have fed me so much on it since I have been hir that I have lost all of my hair from my head and a good share of my teeth."[42] Another complaint about the methods of heroic practice can be found in the letter from Emily Mason to her sister, Catherine Mason Rowland, in 1840. She had been suffering with a "terrible pain" in her face, "the results of cold." "Today," she wrote, "I am threatened with leeching—Don't you envy me having those sweet little worms in my mouth?"[43]

Popular magazines and newspapers joined in a not-so-subtle attack upon the practice of medicine and upon the men who administered it. In 1839, in reporting that two Thomsonians who prescribed only botanical drugs were being tried in New York for the deaths of four smallpox patients, the editor of the New Orleans *Courier* commented: "This is a good commencement, and one which should be extended to others of the medical

---

[40] Brashears, Autobiography, pp. 130–32, cited in Duffy, *Matas History*, II, 354–55.

[41] Duffy, *Matas History*, II, 355.

[42] Charles M. Bull to John Bull, Jr., Detroit, September 13, 1832, November 25, 1832, in C. M. Bull Papers, Burton Historical Collection.

[43] Emily Mason to Catherine Mason Rowland, November 4, 1840, in John T. Mason Papers, Burton Historical Collection.

profession, who, though they treat differently, [have] as many lives to answer for as any of the Thomsonian practitioners."[44] Several years later a Philadelphia editor denounced the "poisoning and surgical butchery" which he said was "common in medicine."[45]

The editor of the *United States Magazine, and Democratic Review* wrote in 1849 that it was seriously asked "whether doctors are really not the final cause of disease." "It is not, of course, to be disputed," he asserted, "that they have been, to no inconsiderable extent, accessory both to the reduction of disease, and—of life itself." In this article, entitled "The Follies of the Faculty," he quoted the French philosopher, D'Alembert, who said that "Nature is fighting with disease; a blind man armed with a club,—that is, the physician,—comes to settle the difference. He first tries to make peace; when he cannot accomplish this, he lifts his club and strikes at random. If he strikes the disease, he kills the disease; if he strikes nature, he kills the patient." The editor concluded that "the less we have to do with physic altogether, the better for longevity."[46] The next issue of that same magazine contained verses from "A Dose of Calomel," a popular song by the Singing Hutchinson Sisters:[47]

> Physicians of the highest rank,
> To pay their fees would need a bank,
> Combine all wisdom, art and skill,
> Science and sense in—*Calomel.*
>
> The man grows worse quite fast indeed!
> Go, call the doctor, ride with speed;
> The doctor comes, like post with mail,
> Doubling his dose of—Calomel!
>
> The man in death begins to groan,
> The fatal job for him is done!
> He dies alas! and sad to tell—
> A sacrifice to—Calomel!

Although perhaps the majority of patients demanded the heroic treatment, as has been shown, there was a ground swell of skepticism both

---

[44] New Orleans *Courier*, January 22, 1839, cited in John Duffy, "The Changing Image of the American Physician," *Journal of the American Medical Association* 200 (April 3, 1967): 32.

[45] *Philadelphia City Item*, November 6, 1858, cited in Richard H. Shryock, *Medicine in America: Historical Essays* (Baltimore, 1966), pp. 150–51.

[46] 22 (March 1848): 215–16.

[47] Ibid. (April, 1848): 360.

within and without the profession. There was a need and growing demand for a moderation of the heroic practices, a need which was to be met by a few orthodox practitioners like Drs. Jacob Bigelow, Samuel Jackson, and Edward H. Barton, and by the growth and development of unorthodox medicine. It was to be first the Thomsonian and then the Homeopath who were to attempt to fill this vacuum formed by the inability of the orthodox profession to provide safe and effective treatments.

II

THE GROWTH OF UNORTHODOX MEDICINE

AN INDIGENOUS FOLK MEDICINE, usually based upon preparations from the local plant life, characterizes every society. The therapeutics of folk medicine are often combined with prayers, objects believed to have some mystical benefit, and other superstitious practices. For instance, in the 1780's, Dr. Peter Turner's recipe for the "Falling Sicknefs or Fitts" was based upon the afterbirth of a first born child. This was sliced and put first "into a pewter platter," then "into a warm oven." The physician would "dry it well & powder it fine," and prescribe a teaspoonful at a time "in French Brandy or sweet wine." The medicine was to be taken according to the doctrine of sacred numbers, that is, "three mornings Successively," then omitted for the following three days, taken again, and so forth, until nine doses had been consumed.[1] The fact that Turner was an orthodox practitioner indicates that the medical profession in the late eighteenth and early nineteenth centuries had a close relationship with domestic and folk medicine.

In rural areas settlers had to be able to treat themselves and their families, for there were few trained physicians available. Although medical knowledge was limited, frontier citizens had to learn enough medicine to treat their common ills. Almanacs gave medical advice, and do-it-yourself handbooks were common. The latter were always popular in an America desperately short of craftsmen and professionals. One of the favorite medical books was William Buchan's *Domestic Medicine, or the Family Physician*, first published in 1769. It went through over twenty editions and was

---

[1] MS in Peter Turner Papers, Library of Congress.

still in print as late as 1840. Buchan was read in a great many colonial households, and his text provided his readers with a handy guide to self-medication.[2]

In 1820 Johann George Hohman published an interesting little compendium of folk remedies, consisting largely of a combination of herbals, superstition, and prayer. For a person who "is falling away," Hohman recommended that he urinate into a pot before sunrise, boil an egg in it, bore three holes in the egg with a needle, and take the egg to a big anthill. The patient would feel relieved as soon as the egg was consumed by the ants. Presumably, the ailment would be transferred to the ants in the process. To "banish Convulsive Fevers," Hohman suggested writing a series of magical letters on a piece of paper, sewing it into a flap of linen, and hanging it around the neck. Interestingly enough, the cure for bleeding was quite effective in minor cases. The patient was instructed to count backwards from fifty to three. After counting forty-eight numbers, clotting should have been completed, and in Hohman's words, "you will be done bleeding."[3] Hohman's remedies were those of German-speaking immigrants, but folk medicine arrived in America with the first settlers.

Housewives of every day and age have been familiar with a number of "sure-fire" domestic remedies. In the early nineteenth century these included peppermint water, catnip tea, onion and beef suet, honey flour, and burgundy pitch. For preventive medicine, America's early homemakers prescribed quassia cups, charms, and anodyne necklaces.[4] One historian has evaluated these domestic remedies and found that in most cases they did no harm and that many reduced pain and proved to be soothing. Furthermore, folk practitioners recognized that some ailments were serious enough to warrant the "fetching" of a trained physician. As compared with the orthodox medicine of the day, however, folk medicine was not necessarily inferior. Although the folk practitioner knew little about the cause of illness, and even less about the mechanics of his remedies, the treatments were the result of ages of trial and error. They frequently succeeded in alleviating pain while allowing nature to provide the healing action.[5]

[2] William Buchan, *Domestic Medicine, or the Family Physician* (Edinburgh, 1769). It went through at least fourteen American editions. Other popular handbooks included two by James Ewell, *The Planter's and Mariner's Medical Companion* (Philadelphia, 1807); and his *Medical Companion, or Family Physician* (3d ed.; Philadelphia, 1816).

[3] Johann G. Hohman, *The Long Lost Friend* (Harrisburg, Pennsylvania, 1820), pp. 9–10, 15, 17.

[4] Fannie Anderson, *Doctors Under Three Flags* (Detroit, 1951), pp. 100–1.

[5] Jo Ann Carrigan, "Early Nineteenth Century Folk Remedies," *Louisiana Folklore Misc.* 1 (January 1960): 43–64.

Correspondence oftentimes included medical advice, which demonstrates the widespread use of domestic medicine. Dudley Woodbridge, for instance, recommended to James Backus the use of "skoak berry, steeped in spirit as a cure for the rheumatism." He had heard of the many cures effected by the skoak, but, he asserted, he had taken it in such massive doses and combined with so many other remedies that he did not know which drug had cured him. In a similar letter a Detroit housewife mentioned the case of a friend who had suffered with a severe sore throat, a cough, and chest pains. "I pursuaded [sic] him to wear a medicated hair skin on his breast," she said, "and made him a bottle of my famous cough mixture and he is now entirely well." Another correspondent, writing nine months later, in 1836, told her grandmother that for a cold she had taken Dr. Grayson's hot pennyroyal tea and barley water. On this occasion, however, the remedy combined with the cold to make her quite sick.[6]

American folk medicine helped pave the way for the development of the first American medical heresy, Thomsonianism. Samuel Thomson, its founder, was born in 1769 in Alstead, New Hampshire. The son of a struggling farmer, his early days were devoted to backbreaking agricultural labor. According to his autobiography, when he was about four years old he first became aware of botanical medicine. There was no physician within ten miles of his father's farm, and an "old lady by the name of Benton" provided medical care. She was a practitioner of folk medicine, treating with drugs, ointments, and other preparations from the local plant life. Young Thomson accompanied her on herb-hunting expeditions. In the process he learned the properties of some of the region's more reliable herbals. He learned, for instance, that when its leaves or stem were chewed, one plant caused profuse salivation and vomiting. Sam was soon daring his unsuspecting young friends to chew on the weed; he enjoyed watching the ensuing discomfort.[7]

Although his interest in medicine continued, Thomson's lack of formal education, along with his inability to afford the cost of apprenticeship, prevented him from following a traditional medical career. Even in the days of apprenticeship, a medical education was still expensive. The corre-

---

[6] Woodbridge to Backus, Marietta, August 23, 1815, in Woodbridge Papers; I. Norwall to C. A. Mason, Detroit, January 15, 1836; E. Mason to E. Moir, New York City, September 26, 1836, and July 17, 1837, in J. T. Mason Papers, Burton Historical Collection.

[7] Samuel Thomson, *A Narrative of the Life and Medical Discoveries of Samuel Thomson, containing an Account of his System of Practice, and the Manner of Curing Disease with Vegetable Medicine, upon a Plan Entirely New* (5th ed.; St. Clairsville, 1829), p. 7

spondence of the Edinburgh-educated Dr. Peter Middleton, a leading New York physician, demonstrates that even in the eighteenth century a poor farm boy could not easily become a doctor. Middleton wrote to the father of a prospective apprentice that since it was inconvenient for the boy to be bound for a number of years, he would be willing to accept ten pounds a year in payment. The Doctor provided that the boy "shall serve me in the way of my businefs faithfully & diligently by Night & by Day; And reveal none of my Secrets in any particular." In return, the physician promised to "instruct him in the different Branches of Medicine as opportunity offers," and to allow him free access to his library.[8]

In an apprenticeship agreement, Job Greene in 1785 contracted to give over Jeremiah Greene to Dr. Peter Turner for a five-year term. The boy was "to be boarded, washed, and mended for, to do no businefs except medical and taking care of his own horse when furnished for himself, to be instructed by the said Doctor Turner in the Practice of Physic and Surgery." In return for this education, Greene promised to give the doctor a total of 250 silver dollars; a $100 down payment, $75 after the second year, and a final $75 after the five years.[9] The cost of such an education was beyond the means of the average American farmer. Moreover, few doctors would accept as an apprentice a boy with Thomson's limited rural background.

Unable to obtain any formal training, young Thomson continued his informal medical education. He learned the properties of a great many plants, and soon he was prescribing for his family and friends. When word of his extraordinary success spread through the rural community his practice grew. At this point in his career, Thomson was performing a public service and not really practicing as a professional physician. He was combining his work as a healer with that of a farmer, and he still depended upon his farm income for support.[10] When, however, his house calls became more numerous, Thomson abandoned the agricultural life for a medical one. His decision to become a full-time doctor was made easier by the fact that he detested manual labor.

Thomson's early success convinced him that he possessed a God-given power to cure through nature. His conviction of a calling enabled him to

[8] Peter Middleton to Charles Clinton, New York City, October 31, 1753, MS in Chicago Historical Society.

[9] Agreement between Job Greene and Peter Turner, October 11, 1785, MS in Turner Papers, Library of Congress.

[10] Thomson, A Narrative, pp. 7–21.

rationalize his inadequate education. As he declared: "I finally concluded to make use of the gift which I thought nature or the God of nature had implanted in me; and if I possessed such a gift, I had no need of learning, for no one can learn that gift."[11] As will be seen later, lack of education was to be one of his best selling-points in an America suspicious of education and wealth.

As a rural physician in New Hampshire, Thomson gradually developed his own theory of the cause of disease. After, in his words, "maturely considering the subject," he came to the conclusion that all animal bodies were composed of four elements—earth, air, fire, and water. Illness was evidence of an imbalance of bodily constituents, normally the result of cold, which he called "lessening the power of heat." In order to cure any disease, the doctor only had to restore the "natural heat" of the body. The system also had to be cleared of obstructions and the body nourished back into health through the use of stimulants. Consciously or not, Thomson was basing his theory upon the traditional Galenic humoral system.[12]

Thomson taught that since disease resulted from the reduction of body heat, in order to cure it was necessary to increase heat, cleanse the system, and provide sustenance. He developed a series of remedies and numbered them accordingly. The stomach would be cleansed by the application of preparation number one, the "emetic herb" with which he had playfully deceived his unsuspecting friends, i.e., lobelia (Indian or wild tobacco), which caused the patient to vomit. It was followed by number two, capsicum (cayenne pepper), which had the ability to increase temperature, at least within the mouth. The Thomsonian practitioners supplemented these with rather intense steam baths, and since their treatment always included these baths, they became known as "steam doctors," or simply, "Steamers." Preparation number three was intended to strengthen the body, to provide both sustenance and stimulation needed to restore the system to equilibrium. It consisted of either myrica (bayberry), nymphaea (pond lily), pinus canadensis (spruce), statica (marsh-rosemary), or rhus glabrum (sumac).[13]

[11] Ibid., pp. 22–28; Samuel Thomson, *New Guide to Health, or Botanic Family Physician, to which is Prefixed the Life and Medical Discoveries of the Author* (Boston, 1835), cited in Alex Berman, "The Thomsonian Movement and its Relation to American Pharmacy and Medicine," *Bulletin of the History of Medicine* 25 (September–October, 1951): 412.

[12] Thomson, *A Narrative*, pp. 30–31.

[13] Ibid., p. 32; Samuel Thomson, *Thomsonian Materia Medica* (12th ed.; Albany, 1841), pp. 58off. See also Philip D. Jordan, "The Secret Six, An Inquiry into the Basic Materia Medica of the Thomsonian System of Botanic Medicine," *Ohio State Archaeological and Historical Quarterly* 52 (October–December 1943): 347–55.

Having developed a system of medical practice, and apparently a successful one, Thomson became an itinerant herbalist. He traveled the roads of
New England, examining those who answered his handbills, selling his
preparations to all who applied for them. Unlike the heroic therapeutics
of the regular physicians, his drugs did not harm the seriously ill patients.
Furthermore, some of his herbals did have medicinal value. Sumac bark, for
example, contains the effective pain killer found in aspirin.

Thomson's success as a healer incurred the jealousy of the local orthodox
practitioners, whose heroic doses and massive bleeding failed to cure disease. His obvious lack of education further added to their distrust. It
seemed impossible that an ignorant farmer could practice effective medicine.
In an attempt to force him out of business, in the fall of 1809 Thomson
was charged with the murder of Ezra Lovett, a patient he had seen in
Massachusetts the previous winter. On January 2 he had been called to see
Lovett, who was "ill of a cold." The herbalist ordered a fire built, put
Lovett's feet on a stove of hot coals, a treatment guaranteed to increase
body temperature. In addition, Thomson wrapped Lovett in a blanket and
"puked him" with a powder in water. During the entire treatment, which
lasted eight agonizing days, Thomson continued to feed Lovett hot "coffee."
All was to no avail. The patient died on January 10.

Thomson was charged with manslaughter by medical malpractice. He was
arrested and locked in a cold, bare, Newburyport jail to await trial. Thomson's friends were so incensed at the horrible prison conditions that they
asked the State Supreme Court to hear the case at a special session. Chief
Justice Theophilus Parsons agreed; the trial began in December of 1809.
The indictment charged the New Hampshire herbalist with murder by the
prescription of lobelia. That accusation was quickly proven to be false.
Although Thomson did use lobelia in his practice, Manasseh Cutler, the
famed botanical physician, examined the evidence and testified that the
"coffee" was marsh-rosemary, a harmless preparation.

The trial proved to be a total farce. Doctor Howe, the leading prosecution witness, was unable to either identify or describe lobelia. That was a
key point in the indictment, since Thomson was accused of prescribing that
"poison." At the point in the proceedings when the "coffee" was alleged
to be lobelia, Judge Alexander Rice, one of Thomson's friends, caused an
uproar in court by eating some of it. The judges and bystanders thought
that he was attempting suicide. When no ill effects were observed, however,
the case for the prosecution was virtually lost. Even Doctor French, Thomson's chief adversary and the one instrumental in drawing up the indictment, admitted under oath that the herbalist had effected cures and that

his drugs were harmless. During the trial the prosecution witnesses continued to discredit Thomson. They testified that he was so totally ignorant of medicine that he called his preparations by such unscientific terms as "well-my-gristle" and "ram-cats." Even that did not convince the justices. The Court found that although the patient had succumbed to unskilled treatment, the doctor was innocent.[14]

In 1813 Thomson traveled to the nation's capital in order to secure patents on his medicines and his system of practice. He said that his primary motive was to "get protection of the government against the machinations of [his] enemies." He undoubtedly sought a monopoly, although he denied that that was the case. Once in Washington, Thomson found that he was expected to provide the botanical names of his preparations. Innocent of such matters, he managed to complete all the forms with the assistance of Dr. Samuel Latham Mitchell, member of the House of Representatives from New York, and on March 3, 1813, he was granted the patents.[15]

Thomson sold family rights to anyone who wanted to learn the botanical practice. For a mere twenty dollars, the applicant was granted the right to prescribe the Thomsonian drugs for himself and his family. The purchase of a right, however, did not include permission to practice medicine on anyone outside the family. It constituted instructions for self-medication rather than a medical education for the commercial practitioner.

Thomsonianism took root in a climate well suited to its development. As noted above, there was already a tradition of domestic medicine. Rural folk expected to treat their own illnesses, and Thomson was enabling them to improve on the type of medical care they were accustomed to. Moreover, the period from the 1820's to the 1840's was characterized by the development of Jacksonian Democracy. That prevailing philosophy emphasized the ability of the individual to do anything he desired, whether it be to learn medicine, to choose his own practitioner, to govern himself, or to be a cavalry officer. It was a time when the successful politician had to appear as the common man, drinking corn cider, living in a log cabin, enjoying the good life. At such a time it was natural for the common man to demand the right to medicate himself. Thomson provided the opportunity. "To make every man his own physician" was his motto.

Following the tradition of William Buchan and Shadrach Ricketson,

14 6 Mass 134; See also Thomson, *A Narrative*, pp. 72–84; and Alexander Wilder, *History of Medicine* (New Sharon, Maine, 1901), pp. 457–59.
15 Thomson, *A Narrative*, pp. 96–98; Wilder, *History of Medicine*, pp. 459–60; Berman, "The Thomsonian Movement," *Bulletin of the History of Medicine* 25 (September–October 1951): 415–16.

Thomson was only one of a long line of self-medication advocates. The earlier ones, however, were trying to overcome the shortage of trained medical men on plantations, aboard ship, and on the frontier. Between the times of Buchan and Ricketson and that of Thomson, a medical profession had emerged. Thomson, however, was calling for a return to the good old days of domestic medicine. With the growth of towns at the end of the eighteenth and the beginning of the nineteenth centuries, rural practice continued to influence much of the nation's health care. Rural folk moving into the towns needed the comfort of self-medication, or at least the assurance of a neighbor-physician. Apparently, they tended to distrust the medical graduate.

LICENSURE

The development of an American medical profession during the last four decades of the eighteenth century brought about an interest in medical licensure. Beginning in 1772, newly established state medical societies secured medical licensure laws granting them the right to examine and license all applicants.[16] Since the societies were organized by orthodox practitioners, it was inevitable that they would refuse to license herbalists and other unconventional practitioners, especially those with little or no education.

In New York the 1806 law provided for the formation of county societies, and it declared that "no person shall commence the practice of physic or surgery within any of the counties of this State until he shall have passed an examination and received a diploma from one of the medical societies." In 1807 the law was amended to provide for a five dollar fine for each month of practice by an unlicensed practitioner. The penalty, however, was not to apply to persons who, although administering medicine, did not pretend to be physicians.

Those using herbs or roots were also exempt. The latter were America's pre-Thomsonian herbalists. In 1827 a new law provided that only licensed physicians could sue to recover payment.

While they did not have to be licensed, the Thomsonians could not depend upon legal process to collect fees from their patients. As a result,

---

[16] Joseph F. Kett, *The Formation of the American Medical Profession* (New Haven, 1968), passim.

they and their supporters began a drive to repeal all medical licensure in New York State. Similar movements appeared in almost every other state. While Joseph Kett has argued that the licensure laws were not particularly oppressive, Alexander Wilder, writing in 1901, insisted that 'irregulars" were prosecuted *en masse*. According to the provisions of the early laws, the Thomsonians should have been relatively satisfied, yet they obviously were so upset that they led the fight to have the laws repealed.[17]

Opposition to the licensure laws included such diverse elements as the Thomsonians, Jacksonian Democrats who opposed all monopolistic legislation, and those who simply disapproved of traditional medical care. The main point at issue was whether the legislature had the right to give the regular profession a monopoly on medical care. The granting of a monopoly implied that the legislature considered the common man incapable of selecting a qualified physician from those claiming competency. In 1841 the antimonopolist Democrats gained control of the New York State legislature. A measure was passed in 1844 repealing the 1827 law and its 1830 amendment. As a result, irregulars as well as quacks legally could practice medicine in New York.[18]

One by one the various states repealed their medical licensure laws, and by 1849 only New Jersey and Louisiana were left with such laws on their books. By the mid-nineteenth century, the practice of medicine was open to any one who considered himself qualified, including many outright quacks and frauds. One effect of repeal, obviously, was to legalize the irregular medical sects which arose in opposition to heroic practice.[19]

HOMEOPATHY

Homeopathy was the sect destined to replace Thomsonianism as America's leading unorthodox medical system. It grew out of the work of the German physician and theorist, Samuel Christian Hahnemann (1755–

---

[17] Compare Kett, *Formation of the Profession* to Wilder, *History of Medicine*, pp. 463–510.

[18] John Duffy, *History of Public Health of New York City* (New York, 1968), I, 234, 474–75; see also Wilder, *History of Medicine*, pp. 463–75, 503–10; and Kett, *Formation of the Profession*, pp. 20–21.

[19] See Wilder, *History of Medicine*, pp. 499–501; *Transactions of the American Medical Association* 2 (Philadelphia, 1849): 326–32; William F. Norwood, *History of Medical Education in the United States before the Civil War* (Philadelphia, 1944), p. 406.

1843).[20] For the purpose of this study, it is not necessary to do more than sketch in bold strokes the life of the founder of homeopathy. The practices he advocated are far more significant than the details of his biography.

Hahnemann was born in Meissen, in Saxony, the son of a porcelain painter. According to tradition his first tutor thought so much of the young man's potential that he volunteered his services. In 1775 Hahnemann went to Leipzig to study medicine, but the city's lack of clinical facilities soon led him to move to Vienna. In 1779 he enrolled at the University of Erlangen, attended the required lectures, defended his thesis, and on August 10 of that same year received his medical degree. As a young physician, he was unhappy with his inability to heal the sick and he became an itinerant, wandering throughout Austria and Germany. He married in 1781, but the obligations of family life did little to encourage success. In order to support himself and his family, Hahnemann gave up medical practice and turned to translating. In 1789 he had returned to Leipzig "desperately poor."

Although disappointing as a medical practitioner, Hahnemann was a prolific writer. Early in his career he flouted the medical practice of the day. Instead of bleeding, blistering, and purging, he prescribed exercise, a nourishing diet, and pure air.[21] His main claim to fame, however, and his major interest, was experimental pharmacology. Hahnemann was interested in determining the exact effects of various drugs upon the human body. Why were they given? What did they do to the system? How did they act to battle disease? In what one historian described as the "absence of any experimental or scientific pharmacology," Hahnemann sought to provide a rational basis for therapeutics.[22] Pharmacology was in such disrepute that the situation was of immediate concern to every physician. Hahnemann complained that if he sent a prescription to ten different pharmacists, invariably he would receive ten different preparations, each having a different effect upon the system.

In 1790 when he translated Cullen's *Materia Medica* into German,

---

[20] The following discussion of the life and work of Hahnemann is derived from Thomas L. Bradford, *Life and Letters of Dr. Samuel Hahnemann* (Philadelphia, 1895); Wilhelm Ameke, *History of Homeopathy; Its Origins; Its Conflicts*, ed. by R. E. Dudgeon (London, 1885); the excellent chapter by Lester King in his *Medical World of the Eighteenth Century* (Chicago, 1958), pp. 157–91; and the chapter on homeopathy in Kett, *Formation of the Profession*, pp. 132–64.

[21] S. Hahnemann, "The Friend of Health," in his *Lesser Writings*, ed. by R. E. Dudgeon (New York, 1852), pp. 170, 182–89, 191–200.

[22] King, *Medical World of the Eighteenth Century*, p. 162.

Hahnemann took the first step toward the formulation of the fundamental law of homeopathy, *similia, similibus, curantur* (let likes be cured by likes). He was intrigued by Cullen's explanation of the influence of cinchona, the "jesuit's bark" which was used as a specific for fever. Cullen had asserted that it was effective mainly because of the "strengthening power it exerts on the stomach." Hahnemann rejected that idea and decided to run what amounted to a controlled experiment in order to determine how the bark actually operated. He took four drachms of cinchona twice a day and noted its effect. His extremities grew cold, his pulse hurried, he began to exhibit the symptoms of fever, the flushed countenance, throbbing head, thirst, and so forth. When he discontinued the drug, the symptoms disappeared and he was "soon quite well." Hahnemann reasoned that cinchona produced the fever, not an unreasonable assumption considering the state of science at the time. The bark could reduce fever, yet it had produced fever in a healthy person. According to the law of *similia* which resulted from this and other experiments, disease could be cured by drugs which produced in a healthy person the symptoms found in those who were ill.

Hahnemann further expanded this theory by investigating a number of other drugs. He recommended experimentation on healthy persons, the so-called "drug-provings" which characterized homeopathic research for the next century and a half. He investigated drug action using pure and simple medicines, so he could determine exactly which drug was causing the symptoms. In his experiments, the subject was given the medication and asked to describe his sensations. From a modern standpoint, it was a haphazard method, but it was an advanced concept for the late eighteenth century.

In seeking to explain how the law of *similia* operated, Hahnemann ended up with a modified form of vitalism. According to his theories, the dose prescribed on the basis of the law of *similia* created in the body an artificial form of the same illness, but one which the body was able to combat. He felt that without assistance, the "vital powers" of the body were helpless in the struggle with disease. Hahnemann compared the body's attempt to drive out illness to military alignments. The "native army" could only defeat the "enemy" with help from "auxiliary troops." The homeopathic dose enabled the vital spirit to defeat illness (the "enemy").[23] Thus, the spiritual being was capable of playing a role in causing material change. This, in effect, meant that to prescribe homeopathically and to believe in its

---

[23] Samuel Hahnemann, *The Chronic Diseases; Their Specific Nature and Homeopathic Treatment* (New York, 1846), IV, 1–3.

efficacy, the physician had to have an intense belief in a God who established natural laws. He also had to believe that there was an interrelationship between the spiritual and material aspects of life. Homeopathic physicians, as a result, then, tended toward Swedenborgianism and Transcendentalism.[24]

Along with the law of *similia*, Hahnemann slowly evolved the second principle of homeopathy, the law of infinitesimals. This law declared that the smaller the dose the more effective in stimulating the vital force. He carried this practice to its extremes. Hahnemann claimed that a dilution as minute as 1/500,000th of a grain, or even 1/1,000,000th of a grain, could be effective, and he called these dilutions "high potencies." Although chemical analysis could detect no reason why such a preparation should have any effect, Hahnemann firmly believed that he had discovered a new law of nature. He asserted that "in illness the body is enormously more sensitive to drugs than in health."[25] To orthodox practitioners, who in many cases were prescribing drugs by the spoonful, Hahnemann's ideas were utterly ridiculous.

In addition to the two main doctrines, Hahnemann set forth a number of other views. For instance, he declared that the efficacy of the infinitesimal dose resulted from the physician's method of preparing his medicine. The vital spirit, he asserted, could not be affected unless in preparation the vial was "succussed." A simple dilution was not sufficient; the vial containing the medicine had to be struck against a leather pad a number of times. Through such a procedure, the drug acquired its ability to affect the vital spirit. In his own words, "Homeopathic *dynamizations* are processes by which the medicinal properties of drugs, which are in a latent state in the crude substance, are excited and enabled to act spiritually (dynamically) upon the vital forces."[26]

Another aspect of homepathy was Hahnemann's declaration that chronic disease was the result of allopathic suppression of psora (the itch) and other external disorders. He argued that such diverse ailments as skin problems, deafness, asthma, and insanity all resulted from medical treatment of the itch.[27] This "discovery" was soon abandoned by many homeo-

---

[24] For a fuller discussion of the interrelationship between homeopathy and philosophy, see Kett, *Formation of the Profession*, pp. 141–55.
[25] King, *Medical World of the Eighteenth Century*, pp. 170–71.
[26] Hahnemann, *Chronic Diseases*, V, pp. v–vi.
[27] Ibid., I, passim.

paths, but, as will be seen, it played a significant role in the ridicule of Hahnemann and homeopathy by the orthodox physicians.

In 1810, still while wandering from place to place, Hahnemann published his most important work, the *Organon of Homoeopathic Medicine.* The following year, he printed the first volume of his *Materia Medica Pura,* the result of all his so-called drug provings. He listed the medicines tested and described the symptoms caused by each. It provided a handy guide for the homeopathic prescriber. The physician could question his patient as to his symptoms, scan records of previous drug-provings to find the same "totality of symptoms," and dispense the correct drug in infinitesimal doses.[28] At this point, Hahnemann had developed a system of medical practice completely at variance with the orthodox practitioners, whom he referred to as "allopaths." He declared that they prescribed drugs not on the basis of *contraria* (drugs opposite in reaction to the symptom), or *similia* (like the symptoms), but *allos,* meaning other basis of prescription. The name which Hahnemann coined—"allopaths"—soon was commonly applied to the regular profession. The orthodox practitioners were not happy over the implication that they practiced according to *any* theory. They liked to think that they were thoroughly scientific and not limited to any particular dogma.

Hahnemann's remaining years are irrelevant for our purposes. Suffice it to say that he died in 1843, a successful and wealthy physician, at the ripe old age of eighty-nine. By that time, homeopathy had spread through Europe and across the Atlantic to the New World. It was here in America that the doctrines of the German theorist were to take root and blossom into a large, fairly well-educated medical sect, one strong enough to encourage serious opposition and important enough to profoundly influence American medical practice.

[28] Samuel Hahnemann, *Organon of Homeopathic Medicine* (2d American ed.; New York, 1843); S. Hahnemann, *Materia Medica Pura,* trans. by R. E. Dudgeon (London, 1880).

III

"HOMEOPATHY, AND ITS KINDRED DELUSIONS"

THE EARLIEST HOMEOPATHS to appear in the United States were Hans B. Gram and his disciple, John F. Gray. Gram, a Danish immigrant, returned to Copenhagen to complete his medical education. As a student, he had heard of homeopathy, and after investigating it he was soon a firm advocate of the new system. In 1825 he once again crossed the Atlantic to settle permanently in New York City. Gram was a successful practitioner, and he began to attract converts to homeopathy. Gray, who studied under Gram in New York, opened his own practice in 1828.

America's homeopathic profession grew steadily, with many physicians who were dissatisfied with orthodox medicine joining the ranks. Through a series of trans-Atlantic letters, for instance, two German immigrants, Henry Detweiler and William Wesselhoeft, learned of the new system of medical practice. Soon, they too were enthusiastically practicing homeopathy. In 1833 Dr. Constantine Hering, destined to be America's leading homeopath, arrived in America. According to tradition, Hering had been commissioned to write a book refuting Hahnemann's work. In the course of his research, however, Hering became convinced of the benefits to be derived from homeopathy. Almost immediately, he became an ardent homeopath.[1]

---

[1] The growth of homeopathy in the United States can be studied through the state histories in William Harvey King, *History of Homeopathy and its Institutions in America*, 4 vols. (New York, 1905); Stephen R. Kirby, *The Introduction and Progress of Homeopathy in the United States* (New York, 1864); Joseph F. Kett, *The Formation of the American Medical Profession*, (New Haven, 1968), pp. 135–40. Biographies of individual homeopaths are available in T. L. Bradford, *The Pioneers of Homeopathy* (Philadelphia, 1897).

From Gram's arrival in 1825 to approximately 1840, homeopathy struggled to maintain itself in two or three states. When Hahnemann's works were translated into English and became better known, in the early 1840's, the system gained both in numbers and influence. Its success in the cholera epidemic from 1848 to 1852 brought added publicity and respectability. It was reported that a great many orthodox practitioners were disappointed with the limited success of their own practices in the face of the cholera outbreak. This led to what one historian described as "a widespread desertion from orthodox ranks." In 1849, apparently directly resulting from the relative homeopathic success during the epidemic, a thousand doctors and laymen joined to organize a homeopathic society in Cincinnati, and the following year, 1850, a homeopathic college was founded in Cleveland. By 1852 homeopathy could claim over 300 adherents in New York State, another 20 in Greater Boston, and 53 in Philadelphia.[2]

By the mid-nineteenth century, the new sect had established medical societies in state after state, and in 1844 the American Institute of Homeopathy was organized as the first national medical society. In addition, homeopathic colleges were being founded to train second generation homeopaths.[3] Before 1860, however, the majority of its practitioners were still orthodox physicians who had abandoned their system in favor of the safer and seemingly more effective Hahnemannian method. A Cleveland newspaper noted in 1849 that among the homeopaths convening in that city were "some who held good position among the Allopathists."[4]

Homeopathy was more of a threat to the medical profession than Thomsonianism had been. In the first place, since many homeopaths were recruited from the regular profession, the gains were made at the expense of orthodox medicine. Nor were its practitioners the uneducated backwoodsmen attracted to Thomsonianism; rather, they were well-educated individuals who had discarded their original methods because of their inadequacy.

Although much more research was done by "regulars," the orthodox research was not directed toward developing a system of medical practice. Homeopathy, on the other hand, was a system based upon investigation and research. On that basis, homeopathy seemed more firmly grounded in scientific experimentation than even the orthodox practice. Its adherents

[2] *North American Homeopathic Journal* 2 (November 1852): 493–96; Kett, *Formation of the American Medical Profession*, p. 138.
[3] See *Medical Century* (Chicago), 2 (July 1, 1894): 305–9.
[4] *Cleveland Daily True Democrat*, May 17, 1849, p. 3, col. 1.

were able to argue that unlike the empiricism of the regulars, who prescribed by trial and error, homeopaths treated their patients according to
a well-grounded system. Interestingly enough, the homeopaths were later
to be excluded from orthodox medicine not because of their educational
background, but rather because of their dogmatism.[5]

Popular magazines of the day differed over the merits of homeopathy,
and, indeed, over the benefits of medicine in general. While some journals
favored the new system, others ridiculed it. A writer in the 1831 *North
American Review* discussed the "Character and Abuses of the Medical
Profession." He noted that although every American believed that his
family doctor was "above suspicion," physicians were the most ridiculed of
the professionals. One of the problems was that the orthodox profession
maintained a "bigoted attachment to authorized modes of practice," and
this made physicians unwilling to test or accept innovations. The author
explained that prejudice determined the "conduct of the medical profession
towards irregular practitioners, and their irregular practices."[6]

In 1848 an article in the *United States Magazine, and Democratic Review* favored homeopathy over orthodoxy, simply because its treatments
were not as harsh as those of the regular profession. The author even put
his feelings into verse:

> The homeopathic system, sir, just suits me to a tittle
> It proves of physic, anyhow, you cannot take too little;
> If it be good in all complaints to take a dose so small,
> It surely must be better still, to take no dose at all.

The writer concluded by consoling the medical profession. Although
doctors drove their patients to an early grave, at least they were not as
callous as the "military chieftains" who placed almost no value upon human
life.[7]

Since the homeopathic doctrine appeared to be totally ridiculous, some
magazines used humor to demolish it. In 1834, the *Select Journal*, for
example, reviewed Hahnemann's *Organon* and John B. Gilchrist's *Practical
Appeal to the Public . . . in Defense of the New System of Physic*. The
reviewer made the most of his opportunity. The brilliant Hahnemann, he

---

[5] See Kett, *Formation of the Profession*, pp. 156–64.
[6] *North American Review* 32 (April 1831): 367ff.
[7] *United States Magazine, and Democratic Review* 22 (May 1848): 418.

said, devoted twelve long years of research and study, to discover that all diseases originated from the "ITCH." The review of the *Organon* was concluded with the comment that Dr. S. Stratton, Hahnemann's editor, "only intended a sly hit at the medical profession, or was indulging his facetious dispositions when he signed himself M.D. Perhaps, indeed, he is a Drum-Major." "Of poor Dr. Gilchrist," he refused to say much. "It would be cruel to deprive him of any little amusement he may find in writing books, but his friends ought to take care that they are not published. Homeopathy may have cured his *bodily* maladies, but ————." [8]

The medical profession, as indicated earlier, was as divided as the popular journals in its early reception of homeopathy. In 1830 the *American Journal of the Medical Sciences* reviewed Hahnemann's *Organon* and two other books on homeopathy. The result was a fair, intelligent discussion.[9] The author was Dr. E. Geddings, a medical professor from Charleston, South Carolina. Geddings noted that the doctrine of *similia* had a long past, with Boerhaave, Sydenham, and Hippocrates all recognizing it in the treatment of specific ailments. Despite its acceptance by the leading clinicians of the past, Geddings believed that Hahnemann was too dogmatic in asserting that *similia* held true in every case and that some day it would become the accepted law of cure. Rather, the South Carolinian asserted that homeopathy might furnish "a means, amongst others, of alleviating human suffering." [10]

He likewise rejected Hahnemann's belief that the physician who sought to learn the cause of disease was wasting his time and energy. Symptoms were all important to Hahnemann, and cause was related to symptom. Geddings denied that the elimination of symptoms would cure disease. "We think that we should be acting with quite as much reason," the professor declared, "in attempting to extinguish the awful heavings of a volcano, by throwing back upon it its ejected lava, or to controul [*sic*] the whirl-wind, or rule the storm, by gathering together the fragments occasioned by their devastating influence." [11]

Despite the shortcomings of homeopathy, Geddings continued, Hahnemann had documented so many cures that either homeopathy had "some foundation in truth," or the "science of medicine is all a hoax." If homeopathy had no basis in truth, he said, "we have been literally poisoning

[8] *Select Journal* 3 (January 1834): 68–72.
[9] *American Journal of the Medical Sciences* 7 (1830): 467–88.
[10] Ibid., pp. 468–71.
[11] Ibid., pp. 473–74

our patients, and sending them out of the world with tortured stomachs and shattered systems." Geddings did not believe that minute doses could have any effect other than "that which their ingestion is calculated to exercise upon the imagination." Yet, he recognized that Hahnemann's success indicated that the medical profession was doing a particularly bad job of treating the sick. The South Carolinian was uncertain whether medicine was a blessing or a curse, but he felt that homeopathy had to qualify as a blessing if its drugs neither upset the stomach nor revolted the imagination.[12]

In 1838 James McNaughton read a paper before the New York State Medical Society. It, too, was a fair evaluation of homeopathy, although the doctor was quick to condemn "charlatanism" practiced in its name. He was particularly incensed over the fact that homeopaths, from Hahnemann to his "lowest" supporter, "Vilified and caricatured" the older system of practice. McNaughton called upon the Society to open the wards of a hospital to an experiment in comparative therapeutics, in order to determine the relative merits of the two systems. He declared that even if homeopathy were quackery, even if the infinitesimal doses were useless, it was "harmless quackery." "If diseases can be removed by mere regimen, and the influence of imagination, with safety to the patient," he said, "it is better and pleasanter to do so, than to disturb the system by powerful remedies." He suggested that the safest method was probably somewhere between the two extremes, between the heroic school, which fought disease to the death, and the homeopathic, which in effect did nothing and let nature provide the healing power.[13]

As can be seen from the writings of Geddings and McNaughton, homeopathy was credited with treating disease in a pleasing manner. During the 1830's the American medical profession was almost totally unfamiliar with the tenets of homeopathy, and until the new sect appeared to threaten the profession, homeopathy was not universally maligned. In 1832 the Medical Society of the County of New York bestowed honorary membership upon Dr. Samuel Hahnemann, the founder of the new system of medical practice. Later, when orthodox medicine felt itself threatened by the increasing popularity of homeopathy, Hahnemann's membership was rescinded.[14] During the late 1830's, however, homeopathy began to come in for some

---

[12] Ibid., p. 488.

[13] James McNaughton, *Annual Address before the New York State Medical Society* (Albany, 1838), pp. 3–32.

[14] Medical Society of the County of New York, *Minutes, 1806–1878* (New York, 1880), I, 509; II, 638.

harsh treatment. A Philadelphia company published William Leo-Wolf's *Remarks on the Abracadabra of the Nineteenth Century*, originally printed in Europe, which purported to be an exposé of the foolishness called homeopathy. At about the same time, David M. Reese, a New Yorker, devoted a chapter to homeopathy in his amusing little book, *Humbugs of New York*.[15]

Some regular practitioners who could clearly see the failings of homeopathy were unable to recognize the inadequacies of their own practice. For instance, in 1840 the *New York Journal of Medicine and Surgery* contained an article which thoroughly condemned homeopathy. The author denied that Hahnemann's discoveries were in any way beneficial. He said that he had tested homeopathic remedies upon himself, and had been unable to perceive any effect from the infinitesimal doses. The writer, however, indicated that he was hardly an objective investigator when he said that homeopathy was too ridiculous to merit point-by-point refutation.[16]

Those physicians who were aware of the inadequacies of heroic medicine, however, were quick to recognize the implications of homeopathy. They may have attacked the new system for its seemingly obvious absurdities, yet at the same time they realized that the homeopath was a successful practitioner because he did not harm the patient. Such commentaries as those of Thomas Blachford, the New York physician,[17] Oliver Wendell Holmes, the Boston poet-physician,[18] and Worthington Hooker, a Connecticut doctor,[19] were in that category. They considered homeopathy absurd, yet they recognized that the lesson to be learned from Hahnemann was that nature provided better medical care than the prevailing system.

As the orthodox profession began to feel more and more threatened by the inroads of homeopathy, bitterness manifested itself in the medical journals. The *Boston Medical and Surgical Journal*, for instance, constantly lamented the fact that some allopaths had adopted the new system. "There is a class of timid, weak-minded physicians," the editor exclaimed, "who

[15] William Leo-Wolf, *Remarks on the Abracadabra of the Nineteenth Century* (Philadelphia, 1835); David M. Reese, *The Humbugs of New York* (New York, 1838), chapter IV. During the 1840's and 1850's allopathic students were subjected to repeated denunciations of homeopathy. For examples, see Robley Dunglison, *On Certain Medical Delusions* (Philadelphia, 1842), and Robert M. Huston, *An Introductory Lecture* (Philadelphia, 1846).

[16] *New York Journal of Medicine and Surgery* 2 (January 1840): 241–47.

[17] Thomas W. Blachford, *Homeopathy Illustrated; An Address first Delivered before the Rensselaer County Medical Society* (Albany, 1851).

[18] Oliver Wendell Holmes, *Homeopathy, and Its Kindred Delusions* (Boston, 1842).

[19] Worthington Hooker, "The Present Mental Attitude and Tendencies of the Medical Profession," *New Englander* 10 (November 1852): 561.

for the sake of enlarging the receipts of practice, or obtaining that which they never had, pretend . . . that they discover plausibility in the theory of homeopathy, and admit that there might be some good in it." "Others," he continued, "boldly dash into the experiment of prescribing little pellicles of pulverized sand . . . although they are as totally ignorant of the fundamental principles of homeopathy as the tribe of Flat Head Indians."[20]

In a following issue, "D.C." expressed his agreement with the editor's opinion. He asserted that there were two kinds of homeopaths. The first were the *"par excellance"*—true disciples of Hahnemann—whom he considered to be "arrant fools, or knaves; generally the latter." The second class he identified as those who renounced orthodoxy for the financial rewards to be gained from prescribing the tiny pills of homeopathy. The latter he refused to acknowledge as "physicians." They should be treated, he insisted, as "dishonest and unprincipled." "They have forfeited all title to respect, and if it were withheld from them we should not see so many trimming their sails to catch the popular breeze."[21]

Dr. E. E. Marcy, an editor of the *North American Homeopathic Journal*, sought to maintain his dignity in the face of these attacks. He urged his fellow homeopaths never to let themselves become involved in character assassination. "Combat principles freely, and meet all novel ideas fairly and honestly, but for the sake of our noble science, let no one . . . give countenance to any one who disgraces his calling by circulating falsehoods and calumny against his brethren who differ from him in opinion." Unfortunately, Marcy himself succumbed to the crescendo of hatred wrought by the attacks upon homeopathy. "Eschew especially the contaminating influence of these sacrilegious wretches, and spurn them beneath your feet as foul and slimy reptiles," he said, "whose breath is poison, and whose touch is pollution."[22] Although the allopaths were bitter in their denunciations of homeopathy, as can be seen from Marcy's comments, it was hardly a one-way affair. Like the Thomsonians, the homeopaths were quick to take advantage of the shortcomings of heroic medicine, emphasizing the "murders" which they claimed were daily being committed at the altar of orthodoxy.[23]

[20] *Boston Medical and Surgical Journal* 24 (March 17, 1841): 97.
[21] Ibid. (March 31, 1841): 139–43.
[22] *North American Homeopathic Journal* 1 (November 1851): 525–26.
[23] See, for instance, E. Bayard, *Homeopathia and Nature against Allopathia and Art* (New York, 1858); Henry Wigand, *The Principles of Homeopathic Practice as Contrasted with those of the Old School of Medicine, or Allopathy* (Boston, 1846); and William Cullen Bryant, *Popular Considerations on Homeopathy* (New York, 1841).

Marcy tried to explain the angry reaction of the regulars to the inroads of homeopathy. He said that selfishness was a human characteristic. "When we contemplate the number of families that are daily abandoning" the allopaths, the New York homeopath declared, "and the continually increasing distrust and abhorrence in which their doctrines and practice are coming to be held, we can readily account for the bitterness of their feelings, and their harmless written and oral ravings."[24]

Homeopaths and allopaths were upset by the fact that the steadily increasing number of allopaths who were enlisting into the ranks of homeopathy tended to combine the two systems. Homeopaths were firmly convinced that the two opposite systems could not be mixed. According to Marcy, "if homeopathy be true, allopathy must be false and pernicious, and *vice versa*."[25] The regular profession, on the other hand, was angered when regularly educated physicians either renounced allopathic medicine or combined it with what was an "absurd" and "ridiculous" system. Since homeopathy seemed so foolish, the orthodox profession decided that converts to the new system were not firm in their beliefs. Rather, they had accepted homeopathy in order to provide their patients a choice of treatment.[26]

The classic and most effective attack upon homeopathy came at the hands of Oliver Wendell Holmes, physician, poet, and medical educator. He first presented his entertaining and enlightening classic, "Homeopathy, and Its Kindred Delusions," in 1842 as a set of two lectures before the Boston Society for the Diffusion of Useful Knowledge. Later that year, it was published and widely disseminated. This pamphlet must be studied in order to fully appreciate the arguments used by the profession against what it considered the "quackery" of homeopathy.

Holmes began his assault upon the citadels of homeopathy by demonstrating that the "miraculous cures" claimed by the advocates of the new system really meant very little. The truth of medical doctrine, according to Holmes, had nothing to do with numbers of cures. In order to prove his contention he described several "kindred delusions" of the past. Like homeopathy, they all had effected "great cures," but again like homeopathy, they rested upon no scientific basis. These delusions included the royal touch for scrofula, weapon salve, tar water, and the Perkins' tractor.

In the first of these, Holmes explained that it was long believed that the monarchs of England had the power to cure the "King's evil," or

---

[24] *North American Homeopathic Journal* 1 (May 1851): 295–96.
[25] Ibid., p. 296.
[26] See *Boston Medical and Surgical Journal* 24 (March 17, 1841): 97.

scrofula (tuberculosis of the lymphatic glands), simply by touching the patient. It was customary for the King to complete the treatment by hanging a gold coin around the neck of the sufferer. Numerous cures were reported, to the extent that blind persons were said to have had their sight restored. Some persons claimed to be cured after only one touch; others required a second application. As Holmes noted, to the modern investigator the belief in the royal touch was complete foolishness. Those who claimed such cures were not suffering with scrofula. Also, the "cured" included those whose maladies were psychological. They believed that their ailments would disappear with the touch, but rather than being cured of scrofula they were relieved of their imagined sicknesses. In other cases, the sick may have been putting the touch upon the King, feigning illness in order to get the gold coin which accompanied the treatment.[27]

Holmes's second illustration of a medical delusion was the curious belief in weapon salve. In medieval days, there was the interesting idea that when a man was injured in combat, he could be cured by the simple application of an ointment. The salve, however, was not applied to the wound. Instead, it was put on the weapon which had inflicted the injury. The wound often healed correctly, as it was carefully washed and bandaged. After the wound was dressed, the weapon was anointed with the salve. Many respectable physicians testified to the benefits of the treatment; many of them reported a number of fabulous "cures." Weapon salve obviously had no medicinal value, yet it was widely hailed.[28]

The third example of a delusion considered by the Boston physician was Bishop Berkeley's tar-water. The Bishop had discovered that when a gallon of water was mixed with a quart of tar, and left for two days, the liquid drained off had great medicinal qualities. Berkeley considered it a cure-all, prescribing it for all types of ailments. Holmes noted that the Bishop had died at the age of seventy. His sudden illness left him no time to "stir up a quart of the panacea." According to the Harvard professor, the tar-water was like homeopathy in that there was no scientific reason for it to succeed. Yet, when patients recovered, the cure was credited to the treatment.[29]

The fourth delusion which Holmes likened to homeopathy was the Perkins' metallic tractor. In 1796 Elisha Perkins, a Connecticut physician, discovered that an object made from two three-inch long pieces of iron

---

[27] Holmes, *Homeopathy, and Its Kindred Delusions*, pp. 1–4.
[28] Ibid., pp. 4–7.
[29] Ibid., pp. 7–10.

and brass alleviated pain when applied to an ache. Perkins was convinced that by rubbing his patients with this object, "the tractor," he was capable of curing rheumatism, inflammation, and tumors. He set out to turn his discovery into a fortune. After patenting his invention, Perkins set out to let the world know of his panacea. Before long, he had effected a great number of "miraculous cures." Like the royal touch, weapon salve, and Berkeley's tar-water, the Perkins tractor was soon to be discarded as useless and relegated to history's antique shelf. At the time, however, it won a number of important converts. Many respectable persons in England and America believed that they had been cured by the tractors.

Holmes noted that like homeopathy and every other "delusion," the advocates of the Perkins tractor were quick to advertise their cures. Moreover, they asserted that they were being treated like Harvey and Jenner. The benefits of their "panacea" were denied by those too ignorant to investigate the truth, or unwilling to renounce their own practices. The latter, of course, would be tantamount to admitting that they had sacrificed hundreds of patients, while all the physician had to do was to apply the tractor, the tar-water, weapon salve, or homeopathy. Advocates of a "delusion," Holmes observed, always compared their persecution to that of Christ, Copernicus, and Galileo, and they considered their opponents akin to the Holy Inquisition.[30]

Having placed homeopathy in the company of the quack, charlatan, and mountebank, Holmes proceeded to examine Hahnemann's doctrines. The Boston physician started with the assertion that if a new doctrine was false, it was "a dangerous, a deadly error." If it did not cure, it would only prevent the sick from undergoing more effective and beneficial treatment. The charlatan who treats cancer may be killing his patients. The time consumed in the cancer treatment may have been better employed in a treatment more likely to succeed. Holmes implied that if homeopathy were false, it should be ruthlessly suppressed. It could only harm patients by keeping them from scientific treatment.

Holmes proceeded to describe the major tenets of homeopathy, the doctrine of *similia*, the infinitesimal dose, the belief that chronic disease results from suppression of the itch, and so forth. Holmes correctly noted that all homeopaths agreed that the law of similars was "the only funda-

[30] Ibid., pp. 10–27; See also Jacques M. Quen, "Elisha Perkins, Physician, Nostrum-Vender, or Charlatan," *Bulletin of the History of Medicine* 37 (March–April 1963): 159–66; and James Harvey Young, *The Toadstool Millionaires* (Princeton, 1961), pp. 20–27.

mental principle in medicine," and that the vast majority of homeopaths administered doses in infinitesimals. He recognized that the "psora" doctrine was ignored by some homeopathic practitioners, "notwithstanding Hahnemann says it cost him twelve years of study and research to establish the fact." Despite the disavowal of the psora doctrine, Holmes was convinced that Hahnemann's word was revered by most homeopaths. He briefly examined homeopathy's major doctrines and found that the *similia* had some validity, but not enough to be considered as the only law of cure.[31]

The doctrine of minute doses did not suffer so mild a fate. Since it was necessary for the pharmacist to throw away 99 per cent of the fluid in preparation of each homeopathic dilution, Holmes calculated that it would take an enormous amount of liquid to continue to the seventeenth dilution. For instance, for the first dilution, 100 drops of alcohol would be needed (to be more correct, it should be 99). Since one drop of the mixture would be mixed with another 100 drops, it would take 10,000 drops to complete the second dilution. Holmes was wrong on this point. It was only necessary to have another 100 drops to have one preparation at the second dilution. In any case, he figured that by the seventeenth dilution, the contents of "ten thousand Adriatic Seas" would be needed. Ridiculing homeopathy even further, he declared that one drop of medicine, if carried to high potencies, would provide more than five billion doses to every individual who ever lived on earth.[32] Having thus disposed of the doctrine of infinitesimals, he turned his weapon upon Hahnemann's most vulnerable doctrine, the "psora."

When a German physician discovers that the itch is the "great scourge of mankind, the cause of their severest bodily and mental calamities, cancer and consumption, idiocy and madness." Holmes exclaimed, "does it not seem as if the very soil upon which we stand, was dissolving into chaos, over the earthquake heaving of discovery?" Further, when one man claims to have discovered the three independent laws, as "remote from each other, as the discovery of the law of gravitation, the invention of printing, and that of the mariner's compass," the question naturally arises, "is not this man deceiving himself, or trying to deceive others?"[33]

Holmes began his demolition of Hahnemann's drug-provings after having disposed of the itch. He listed the symptoms which Hahnemann's

[31] Holmes, *Homeopathy, and Its Kindred Delusions*, pp. 29, 34–37.
[32] Ibid., pp. 37–40.
[33] Ibid., pp. 40–41.

subjects had ascribed to the various drugs. Then he asserted that they seemed to be scarcely grounded in fact. To cite an example, Holmes noted that according to Hahnemann, muriatic acid produced the following symptoms: sighing, pimples, "after having written a long time with the back a little bent over, violent pain in the back and shoulder-blades, as if from a strain," dreams "which are not remembered,—disposition to mental dejection,—wakefulness before and after midnight." He suggested that Hahnemann had ascribed the sensations encountered in daily life to the drug under investigation. Furthermore, he noted that the eminent Paris allopath, Andral, had investigated the drug-provings, and found that he could not reproduce the symptoms listed by Hahnemann. Holmes concluded that through common sense and Andral's scientific study, drug-provings were hardly worthy of confidence.[34]

The Boston poet-physician attempted to verify Hahnemann's references, but he was unable to find many of them. Of the few he could locate, he discovered "two to be wrongly quoted, one of them being a gross misrepresentation." Hahnemann had used ancient authorities to demonstrate that the doctrine of *similia* was recognized in specific ailments by reputable clinicians of the past. Holmes's findings cast doubt upon Hahnemann's objectivity.[35]

Holmes went on to examine the problem of statistics. Many homeopaths claimed that their system was more effective than the orthodox practices. For instance, they argued that during cholera epidemics homeopathy had proved far superior to heroic treatment. They cited statistics which showed that homeopathic hospitals had lower mortality rates than their allopathic counterparts. Holmes swept into battle with the homeopathic statisticians. First, he noted that statistics were always unreliable. In order to compare mortality rates, one must be certain than diagnosis was the same. In one hospital, or to one physician, any illness might be considered cholera, especially during an epidemic. Poor diagnosis would improve the percentage of cure, but it would mean nothing other than that the doctors had disagreed. In addition to the problem of diagnosis, Holmes said that other factors made it impossible to compare hospital mortality rates. These factors included type of disease admitted, location of the institution, and the season of the year.

As the system of treatment was not the sole determinant, then, com-

---

34 Ibid., pp. 41–45.
35 Holmes, *Homeopathy, and Its Kindred Delusions*, pp. 45–49.

parative rates could not be an accurate test of the merits of either system. For instance, Pierre Louis, the Paris physician, was noted for his treatment of consumption. As a result, the wards of the Hospital de la Pitié were usually filled to overflowing with patients in the last stages of that disease. Their eventual deaths would add to the hospital's mortality rate, but it meant very little. Holmes even suggested that the institutions "enjoying, to the highest degree, the confidence of the community, will lose the largest proportion of their patients." Persons suffering from severe disorders would go to the better hospitals, and their passing would raise the mortality rate of a fine institution. On the other hand, "the subjects of trifling maladies, and mere troublesome symptoms, amuse themselves to any extent among the fancy practitioners," among which, of course, Holmes included the homeopaths. He noted that when a Doctor Muhlenbein stated that as a homeopath the mortality rate among his patients was only one per cent, whereas when he was an allopath, it was 6 per cent, it simply indicates that when his patients are "*seriously* sick," they take "good care not to send for Dr. Muhlenbein!" [36]

The real problem in evaluating the merits of homeopathy and other "delusions," according to Holmes, was that the vast majority of patients recover under *any* system. He asserted that 90 per cent of the cases commonly seen by a physician "would recover, sooner or later, with more or less difficulty, provided nothing were done to interfere seriously with the efforts of nature." If a doctor gave a placebo to 100 patients, 90 of them would get better. In the language of the charlatan, the treatment "cured" 90 per cent. That is the precise reason why witch doctors in primitive societies gain the confidence of their patients. By prayer or ritual dances, they cured nine of every ten patients. Thus, Holmes said, even the so-called "scientific" claims of reputable physicians can be seriously questioned. The remedy may have had nothing at all to do with the so-called "cure." Through this line of reasoning, he was able to cast doubt upon the claims of the homeopaths who were reporting "miraculous cures." [37]

Holmes concluded with a number of predictions on the future of homeopathy. First, "the confidence of the few believers in this delusion will never survive the loss of friends who may die of any acute disease, under a treatment such as that prescribed by Homeopathy." Second, "after its novelty has worn out, the ardent and capricious individuals who constitute

[36] Ibid., pp. 50–52.
[37] Ibid., pp. 52–55.

the most prominent class of its patrons will return to visible doses, were it only for the sake of a change." Third, "the semi-Homeopathic practitioner will gradually withdraw from the rotten half of his business and try to make the public forget his connection with it." Finally, "the ultra Homeopathist will either recant and try to rejoin the medical profession; or he will embrace some newer and if possible equally extravagant doctrine; or he will stick to his colors and go down with his sinking doctrine." "Very few will pursue the course last mentioned," Holmes predicted.[38]

The *Christian Examiner*, a Boston magazine, reviewed Holmes's essay. The editor declared that although homeopathy seemed foolish, it deserved a fair trial. If it were more successful than orthodoxy, he asserted, it indicated that the weapons of the regular profession were inadequate. "Gladly would we see banished from the sick chamber the nauseous drugs, the offensive draughts, the pill, the powder, the potion, and all the painful and debilitating expedients of our present system, in favor of the mild and gentle measures of Homeopathy."[39]

One homeopath rushed for pen and paper to defend his system against the attack by Dr. Holmes. In an extraordinarily well-written pamphlet, Dr. A. H. Okie employed enough wit and logic to repel the onslaught by the Boston physician. First, Okie sought to answer the allegation that homeopathy was curing through the use of suggestion. He claimed that only after a long series of successful experiments would the allopaths have the right to proclaim the "influence of imagination and the nullity of Homeopathy as a positive system." "But then," he urged the regular physician to "throw aside the lancet, the scarificator, and the leech; . . . cure your patients by *imagination*, and you will have arrived at the very acme of the art of healing." Psychosomatic medicine, in any case, was inadequate to explain the successes of homeopathy. Okie reported that he had cured unconscious patients as well as babies and animals. Obviously those were groups in which suggestion would have little influence.[40]

Okie was particularly upset over the fact that, although Holmes admitted that he had not tried homeopathic prescribing, he was critical of it. In effect, then, Holmes was saying that whereas "many persons, having written in favor of Homeopathy without understanding it, I a medical man, intend to enlighten the world upon a subject, of which I am totally ignorant

[38] Ibid., pp. 69–70.
[39] *Christian Examiner* 32 (May 1842): 245–72.
[40] A. H. Okie, *Homeopathy; with Particular Reference to a Lecture by O. W. Holmes, M.D.* (Boston, 1842), pp. iii–iv.

practically." Rather than heaping ridicule upon ridicule, Okie insisted that Holmes should have investigated the scientific claims of the new system.[41] He cited case after case to indicate that homeopathy *was* successful. He also showed that the orthodox profession could not even agree upon the cause of disease. He reminded the Bostonian that the orthodox profession was completely at a loss when faced with epidemic disease. Was it brought on by miasma? Little animals? Vitiated atmosphere? What, he asked, was the cause of disease? Since there was such widespread disagreement as to the exact causation, Okie asked, what could be wrong with considering illness as a group of symptoms?[42]

Okie disputed the claim that drug-proving was haphazard and irrelevant to the practice of medicine. It was more foolish, he asserted, to administer remedies without any knowledge of their effects, than to experiment with them on healthy persons. Okie observed that if a healthy person could not describe the effect of a remedy, "what are you to expect from a sick person?" Perhaps drug-proving was unscientific, he said, but was it not more unscientific to prescribe drugs without knowing what the effect would be?[43]

Holmes had declared that nonprofessionals had no right to participate in medical disputes, since they had no basis for judging the truth of medical theory. Okie replied that throughout medical history, the profession had subscribed to theories and practices which have been proved to be completely false. First, the humoralists had claimed that disease was the result of body fluids. That had been discarded as false. Then, Cullen provided the basis for the antiphlogistic regimen—bleeding and purging. Now this was slowly being abandoned by the profession. If physicians were unable to judge theories, indeed, if they had held to false practices for centuries on end, why should the patients be denied the opportunity to judge on the basis of success and failure? Okie asked if physicians should "enjoy the privilege of slaughtering us without being called to account for it?" "What would have become of the Reformation," he asked rhetorically, "had not the laity taken part in it?" If it were left to the theologians, he asserted, "Luther would have been burnt at the stake" and Protestantism would have been stillborn.[44]

Okie had capably defended his colleagues against the sarcasm of Holmes.

[41] Ibid., pp. 6–8.
[42] Ibid., pp. 8–20.
[43] Ibid., pp. 21–23.
[44] Ibid., pp. 25–27.

Unfortunately for homeopathy, the pamphlet by Holmes was given wide publicity, due to the eminence of the author, whereas the reply by Okie was apparently disregarded. Yet, Okie had emphasized the alternatives to homeopathy. Those alternatives, as practiced by the medical profession, were bleeding, blistering, purging, cupping, and sweating. The alternative to drug-proving, he said, was the dispensing of drugs without knowing the effect. Likewise, he asserted that the alternative to the judging of medical theory by the laity was the continuing disagreement by the profession. While the physicians were arguing over the cause of disease, and while the profession had historically lent its credence to false theories, he suggested that perhaps the nonprofessional could better judge medicine on the basis of success. Above all, Okie had shown that there *was* some basis for homeopathic law. Rather than devoting his time to writing satire, he said, Holmes would have done better to investigate and experiment with the practices of the new system.

The editor of the *Boston Medical and Surgical Journal* was surprised to see such sophisticated replies as those by Okie and his homeopathic colleagues, Neidhard and Wesselhoeft, who also defended their practice against its first major attack.[45] "The authors give evidence of being candid, sincere, high-minded men, who will quarrel genteely." Dr. Okie, the editor said, "evidently winces under the thumb-screwing of Dr. Holmes." Yet, in his attempt to defend homeopathy, the editor said that Okie "exhibits more ingenuity than was expected when we commenced reading the review to which he appended his name." "Much as we individually question the pretended merits of homeopathy, justice requires that it should be acknowledged that Dr. O. shows himself a person of extensive reading, an inquirer after truth, and a devoted worshipper at the shrine of Hahnemann." The latter attribute, the editor asserted, was "the only fault that any one could find with him." The editor continued to note that since homeopathy had such able and sincere defenders, at least these few should be accepted as men of science.[46] His colleagues, however, were not so willing to accept these "self-deceived" men as men of science. Rather, they continued to consider them mountebanks and charlatans, men who were willing to rely upon the credulity of their patients in order to amass fortunes.

[45] For other homeopathic replies to Holmes, see Charles Neidhard, *An Answer to the Homeopathic Delusions of Dr. Oliver Wendell Holmes* (Philadelphia, 1842); and Robert Wesselhoeft, *Some Remarks on Dr. O. W. Holmes's Lectures on Homeopathy and its Kindred Delusions* (Boston, 1842).

[46] *Boston Medical and Surgical Journal* 27 (August 24, 1842): 56–57; (September 7, 1842): 86–87.

In 1851 the essay which won the Fiske Award of the Rhode Island Medical Society came off the presses. The prize was given for the best dissertation upon the subject: "Homeopathy, So-called, Its History and Refutation." The winning author was Dr. Worthington Hooker, a leading member of the Connecticut medical profession.[47] The previous year, he had won the same award for the best essay on "the History of Medical Delusions of the Present and Former Times."[48] Hooker sought to apply the rules of evidence to medical practice in order to expose the errors and delusions of homeopathy. In itself, the fact that a prize was given for the best attack upon homeopathy indicates the state of relations between the two schools of thought. Yet, Hooker's work is valuable in its own right, and as such it is worthy of examination.

Before beginning his "refutation of the homeopathic delusion," the Connecticut physician warned his readers not to become upset if he resorted to ridicule. "When things are exceedingly laughable," he declared, it was "a little unreasonable to demand of us an imperturbable gravity. When Homeopathy conjures up its ridiculous fantasies to play before us like so many harlequins, it is hard to be denied the privilege of laughing at them." Again, "if a little pleasantry suffice to demolish an error, it surely is an unnecessary waste of power to attack it with strong and sober argument."[49]

Hooker related the story of Hahnemann's life, and he was surprisingly accurate. After the historical presentation, however, he asserted that since Hahnemann had openly sold "secret nostrums" early in life, he was obviously not only a "mercenary quack" but also a dishonest one. From this inauspicious start, the founder of homeopathy developed a system of practice which, Hooker said, was "so absurd, that it seems almost a waste of time and effort to go through a formal refutation of it."[50]

Hooker used mathematics to demonstrate that the theory of infinitesimals was so insane that only a madman or a knave would consider it a medical law. One grain of any drug, if brought to high potency, he declared, would "be sufficient to supply all the Homeopathic physicians in the world with all which they would want to use . . . in a whole year." To illustrate his point, Hooker quoted the following poem:

---

[47] Worthington Hooker, *Homeopathy: An Examination of its Doctrines and Evidences* (New York, 1851).

[48] Worthington Hooker, *Lessons from the History of Medical Delusions* (New York, 1850).

[49] Hooker, *Homeopathy*, pp. vii–viii.

[50] Ibid., pp. ix, 1–14.

Take a little rum,
the less you take the better;
Pour it in the lakes
of Wener and of Wetter.

Dip a spoonful out,
mind you don't get groggy;
Pour it in the lake
Winnipissiogee.

Stir the mixture well,
lest it prove inferior;
Then put half a drop
into Lake Superior.

Every other day,
take a drop of water;
You'll be better soon,
or at least you ought to.[51]

Hooker moved from mathematics to logic in order to disprove homeopathy. First, he said that the *similia* was not the "sole law of cure." If it were, if opium produced insensibility in the healthy, it would always have to cure it in the sick. Further, if it were the "sole law," cures could be effected in no other way. Thus, no drug except one based upon drug-provings could cure pleurisy. Since every allopath knew, however, that bleeding almost invariably cured that ailment, the homeopathic law could not be the "sole law of cure."[52]

The Connecticut physician followed Holmes in arguing that the fact that people had been "restored to health" while taking homeopathic remedies did not necessarily mean that the remedy provided the cure. He saw this as the primary reason for the success of all such "delusions and quackery." Hooker was not impressed by the fact that many homeopaths were men who had been converted from orthodoxy. If they were poor allopaths, of course they would get better results by treating homeopathically. At least they would not kill their weaker patients. If they were bad allopaths, their success as homeopaths would only indicate that homeopathy was "better than *bad* allopathy."[53] Hooker implied that bleeding, purging, and over-dosing was bad allopathy, and he suggested that homeopathy gained its converts from practitioners of that type of medicine.

[51] Ibid., pp. 21–25.
[52] Ibid., pp. 54–58.
[53] Ibid., pp. 95–100.

Hooker made a valid point when he noted that like all "delusions," homeopathy attracted a number of chronic cases. The chronically ill, he said, were "always getting better, but never get well." Further, those patients did better with little medicine than with a lot. Since the chronically ill are always seeking a panacea, they provide the bulk of cases for all new systems of practice.[54]

Hooker concluded his essay with an analysis of the character of Samuel Hahnemann. The founder of homeopathy, he said, was sincere in his beliefs, although "morally he was a *cheat*." Blinded by the facts of a few cases, he developed a system which was shallow in its foundation and totally unscientific. Hooker called Hahnemann a "medical fanatic," and his system "scientific insanity." He said that his "Psoric theory, the climax of all medical absurdities, shows a height of delusion which has seldom been reached by the human mind." According to Hooker, far from being a scientist, Hahnemann was illogical, inconsistent, and one who confused supposition for fact. "The advocates of Homeopathy, like its founder, are dreamers, and not thinkers." Yet, Hooker recognized that the "same principles of evidence which reject Homoeopathic observation as inconclusive and false, must, if rigidly applied, reject a large portion of the observations contained in the annals of medicine." Homeopathy had demonstrated that the healing power of nature was stronger than that of the heroic practices. Now, Hooker declared, medicine must learn to harness that power. "It is in this way," he said, "that the most absurd of all medical delusions may be made to do essential service to the cause of science and humanity."[55]

Dr. J. T. Curtis, an editor of the *North American Homeopathic Journal*, rushed to defend homeopathy against the assaults by Hooker and the other allopaths who were condemning the new system. In a review of Hooker's prize-winning essay, Curtis suggested that Hooker give homeopathy a fair trial. "Far better had it been for him," the New York homeopath declared, "had he, like the Knight of La Mancha decreed his barber's basin (take note of the history of venesection!) to be an excellent helmet and spared himself a joust for which his pasteboard armor so ill befits him."[56]

It was quite easy for Holmes and Hooker to ridicule homeopathy. Yet, until the orthodox profession knew exactly where orthodoxy was inade-

[54] Hooker, *Homeopathy*, p. 104.
[55] Ibid., pp. 118–24, 138–39.
[56] *North American Homeopathic Journal* 2 (February 1852): 82–93.

quate, and could alter its methods, homeopathy would survive and gain the confidence of the people. Patients were not concerned with medical theory. The sick wanted to be cured, and were willing to use whatever method promised success. Moreover, by arguing that homeopathy was too absurd and ridiculous to deserve refutation, the orthodox profession was closing its mind to a possible improvement in medical practice. Simply because something *seemed* ridiculous did not necessarily mean that it *was* absurd or ridiculous. Homeopathy could not be destroyed by ridicule. Until allopathic medicine was able to provide a more effective cure, homeopathy would continue to gain adherents and to increase in popularity.

IV

THE CONSULTATION CLAUSE

THE REPEAL of America's medical licensure laws opened the profession to all who claimed to be physicians. As noted earlier, the "democratic" impulse was one factor in the movement to abandon those statutes. In his interesting little book, *The Humbugs of New York,* David M. Reese stated the principles of Jacksonian democracy as applied to medicine. He asserted that "the people regard it among their vested rights to buy and swallow such physick, as they in their sovereign will and pleasure shall determine; and in this free country, the democracy denounce all restrictions upon quackery as wicked monopolies for the benefit of physicians." [1] The laws which had established medical societies and authorized them to examine all applicants were soon erased from the books. To the common man, it was a triumph of democracy.

In 1848 the editor of the *Ohio Medical and Surgical Journal* complained not only that it was too easy to become a doctor but also that the public accepted every pretender without question. Anyone who could "raise a pair of saddlebags and fill it with 'roots' and 'arbs,'" was considered qualified as a physician. [2] Two years later, in 1850, Lemuel Shattuck, one of America's pioneering sanitationists, agreed that the medical profession was being crowded with incompetents. He declared in his celebrated *Report of the Sanitary Commission of Massachusetts* that any one, "male or female, learned or ignorant, an honest man or a knave, can assume the name of

---

[1] David M. Reese, *The Humbugs of New York* (New York, 1838), p. 124.
[2] *Ohio Medical and Surgical Journal* 1 (September 1848): 101.

physician, and 'practice' upon any one, to cure or to kill, as either may happen, without accountability. It's a free country!"[3]

Although the demand to repeal the licensure laws came from the general public as well as from those who insisted upon their "right" to be a physician, the medical profession must share in the responsibility. Indeed, conditions were so scandalous within the profession that it is easy to understand why the community lost its respect for the doctor. America's westward expansion increased the demand for physicians on the frontier, and medical colleges were established in order to supply the territories and new states. During the period from 1830 to 1850, the number of medical schools more than doubled. Those colleges had no endowment and had to rely upon tuition fees for financial support. The schools which could attract the largest number of students would be the most prosperous. The situation finally resulted in a vigorous competition for students. The colleges tried to increase enrollment by lowering admission standards, shortening the term of study, and reducing graduation requirements. As a result, the profession became flooded with men who in many cases could barely read or write.[4]

Besides the influx of inferior physicians, the profession was constantly embarrassed by the publicized rivalries within medical faculties and societies. In 1826, for instance, a dispute within the College of Physicians and Surgeons, in New York City, resulted in the release of the entire faculty and the complete reorganization of the college.[5] Although that was an extreme case, dissension was rife among the various faculties. The main points at issue were control over appointments, nominations for the leading chairs, and professional jealousy. Quarrels often resulted in pamphlet wars which were hardly complimentary to the profession. In addition, doctors publicly disagreed with their colleagues on such matters as the causes of disease and the merits of various treatments.[6] Another source of popular disapproval of the profession was the harsh orthodox treatment. The aver-

[3] Lemuel Shattuck, *Report of the Sanitary Commission of Massachusetts, 1850* (Cambridge, 1948), p. 58, cited in James H. Young, "American Medical Quackery in the Age of the Common Man," *Mississippi Valley Historical Review* 47 (March 1961): 583.

[4] Donald E. Konold, *History of American Medical Ethics, 1847–1912* (Madison, 1962), pp. 4–5; Nathan Smith Davis, *History of the American Medical Association, from Its Organization up to January, 1855* (Philadelphia, 1855), p. 19.

[5] Konold, *History of American Medical Ethics*, p. 5.

[6] For example, see Kett, *The Formation of the American Medical Profession* (New Haven, 1968), pp. 59–64, 79–94; and Richard H. Shryock, "Public Relations of the Medical Profession in Great Britain and the United States: 1600–1870," *Annals of Medical History*, n.s., 2 (May 1930): 308–39.

age allopath, as noted above, bled to excess, administered large doses of calomel and opium, and, the result, if not lethal, often lengthened the time of illness.

When medical societies began to establish fee lists, however, the public really became aroused. It was bad enough to inflict a harsh and brutal treatment upon the patient; it was even worse to increase the price. Although the "fee bills" were intended to eliminate underbidding and to establish minimum rates which could easily be paid, the public saw it as an attempt to prevent competition. Moreover, the establishment of fees was contrary to Jacksonian democracy, which was opposed to all monopolistic practices. In 1833 when a group of doctors in the District of Columbia organized to regulate rates, the citizens were so outraged that they held a series of indignation meetings and tried to convince outside physicians to relocate in the area. Of course, newcomers would charge lower rates than the fee bill provided.[7]

In summary, then, all those factors, the state of medical practice, the faculty disputes, the inability of the doctors to agree upon diagnosis and treatment, the inferior physicians annually "turned loose" upon the community, and the monopolistic tendencies of the profession, combined to reduce the prestige and influence of the physician. These help to explain the widespread demand to repeal the licensure laws, which would break the monopoly of orthodox medicine.

In 1849 Dr. Worthington Hooker, who later was to denounce homeopathy, examined the relationship between physician and society. According to his analysis, the major problem was quackery and the "spirit of Quackery" which motivated "quite a large proportion of the profession." Rather than consisting of honorable men seeking to aid humanity, Hooker insisted that the profession was crowded with those who sought only fame and fortune.[8] It was common for the physician to advertise his successes, publish testimonials to his skill, and promise cures. Instead of comforting the desperately ill, many doctors made "gloomy prognostications" in order to magnify their own importance and mitigate the blame for their failure to cure such difficult cases. If his ministrations were successful, however, he was a master craftsman who had wrested his patient from the jaws of death.[9]

[7] See Konold, *History of American Medical Ethics*, p. 7.
[8] Worthington Hooker, *Physician and Patient; or a Practical View of the Mutual Duties, Relations and Interests of the Medical Profession and the Community* (New York, 1849), pp. 250–52.
[9] Ibid., pp. 251–52.

In order to strike "a most effectual blow" against such quackery, the Connecticut physician urged his colleagues to purge the incompetents from their ranks. If doctors could organize to eliminate the orthodox "quacks," the profession could "present a bold, unbroken front in its warfare with empiricism." [10] The purge would be made permanent by a reform of medical education. Hooker asserted that the lower the standard of education, the greater the number of "ignorant pretenders." [11]

Hooker's analysis was fully in line with professional thought. America's doctors sought to regain their lost prestige and influence through improved education. In 1835 the faculty of the Medical College of Georgia called for a convention to discuss the need for reform. The proposal was almost completely disregarded by representatives of the various colleges, and no meeting was held. Four years later, in 1839, the Medical Society of the State of New York debated ways to improve the caliber of the orthodox profession. During the discussion Dr. John McCall, of Utica, proposed that the Society call a "National Medical Convention" at Philadelphia in 1840. Three delegates from each state society and one from each medical college were to gather to find some way to regain lost prestige. Unfortunately for the cause of reform, not one society or college replied to the invitation. In 1844 the New York Society once again discussed the problem. Resolutions were offered which condemned the four-month course of study as too short to cover adequately all aspects of medical science, and which declared that the standards of both preliminary and medical education were too low to ensure the graduation of qualified practitioners.[12]

In 1845 the Society once again discussed medical education. The profession was so disorganized, so ineffectual, and so besotted with incompetents that some physicians even implied that the public was correct in refusing to allow it to control its own destiny. The New York Society demonstrated the extent of the problem when a resolution to raise the standards of the local schools was bitterly opposed. It was argued that higher standards of education in one state would drive prospective students to states with lower standards. Setting high standards in one state, then, would only decrease enrollment in that state. Dr. Alden March, an Albany physician, suggested to Dr. Nathan Smith Davis, the leader in the fight to improve education, that the objections might be overcome if *all* the colleges could be induced

[10] Ibid., pp. 250–53.
[11] Ibid., p. 253.
[12] Davis, *History of the American Medical Association*, pp. 19–21. Morris Fishbein, *A History of the American Medical Association* (Philadelphia and London, 1947) follows the Davis account.

to act in unison. If every American school raised its standards, the New York colleges would not hesitate to act. When Davis proposed a resolution calling for a convention to set national standards, the Society agreed to hold one in May of 1846.[13]

Now that a convention had been called, the Philadelphia schools were reluctant to co-operate with their competitors from New York. The Philadelphia faculties believed that rather than intending to improve education the convention was an attempt to advertise the local schools. On March 11, 1846, Professor Martyn Paine, of the medical department of New York University, "defended" the profession in a speech which altered the course of events. Unwittingly, Paine helped to dispel the idea that the advocates of reform were motivated by selfishness. Davis and the State Society, he declared, had defamed the profession in order to have an excuse to call a convention, the true intention of which was to "cripple the College" by raising standards. Paine and his colleagues apparently wanted to block the convention because, as Davis later wrote, "it originated in a State Society . . . of whose influence they were jealous." When Dr. Robert M. Huston, of the Jefferson Medical College, read Paine's address he realized that the convention *was* a sincere attempt to improve medical education. He convinced the Philadelphia County Medical Society to send twelve delegates to the New York meeting. This episode is indicative of the problems which beset the profession.[14]

The first actions of the fledgling American Medical Association were taken at that 1846 convention. It was resolved "That it is expedient for the medical profession of the United States to institute a *National Medical Association* for the protection of their interests, for the maintenance of their knowledge and the extension of their usefulness." The delegates agreed that there should be standard and improved requirements for the medical degree, that every student should possess a suitable preliminary education, and that the entire profession should be governed by a code of ethics.[15]

In 1847 the committee which had been appointed to formulate the code of ethics reported that it had prepared a code based upon that written in 1796 by the English physician Thomas Percival.[16] The code, adopted in

[13] Davis, *History of the A.M.A.*, pp. 22–23.
[14] Ibid., pp. 24, 28–31.
[15] Ibid., p. 34; *Proceedings of the National Medical Conventions Held in New York, May, 1846, and in Philadelphia, May, 1847* (Philadelphia, 1847), pp. 17–21.
[16] Konold, *History of American Medical Ethics*, pp. 9–13.

May of 1847, included the so-called "consultation clause," which pertained to relations between orthodoxy and the medical sects. The consultation clause asserted that the good of the patient was the sole object of consultations between two or more physicians. Furthermore, no intelligent, licensed practitioner of good moral and professional standard, should either be excluded from fellowship, or his aid refused in consultation. The code continued, however, by insisting that "no one can be considered as a regular practitioner, or a fit associate in consultation, whose practice is based upon an exclusive dogma, to the rejection of the accumulated experience of the profession." [17] No homeopath, then, could consult with an orthodox physician, even if the patient requested such a meeting. Likewise, no regular practitioner could come to the aid of a patient whose doctor was a homeopath, unless the homeopath was first dismissed from the case, regardless of how desperately ill the patient, or how necessary the consultation.

There is evidence to indicate that the struggle against homeopathy was a major factor in the formation of the American Medical Association. In 1883 Dr. Henry G. Piffard, one of America's early dermatologists, wrote that the A.M.A. was established by the orthodox profession in reaction to the "evils of sectarian medicine." According to Piffard, in 1842 the Orange County Medical Society expelled a Doctor Paine, a homeopath. Paine's friends convinced the New York State Legislature to withdraw the power to license from the county societies. That, in turn, resulted in the formation of clubs dedicated to the destruction of homeopathy. "It seemed probable," Piffard declared, that "the most effective blow would be given to the newborn heresy, if the profession as a whole combined against it. It seemed necessary that the homeopaths as a body should be absolutely excommunicated from professional recognition and intercourse, and that the public at large should know it. In the code of ethics, and especially in the consultation clause, this sentiment crystallized." [18]

There is much more evidence, however, to indicate that although the development of homeopathy was one reason for the formation of the A.M.A., the main impetus came from natural forces in social and medical thought. First of all, the fight to repeal the New York licensure law was led not by homeopaths, but by Thomsonians. This can be seen from the fact that the followers of Samuel Thomson drafted the petition opposing the

---

[17] *Code of Ethics of the American Medical Association, adopted May, 1847* (Philadelphia, 1848), pp. 18–19.

[18] Henry G. Piffard, "The Status of the Medical Profession in the State of New York," *New York Medical Journal* 37 (April 14, 1883): 401.

law, and the signed petitions were so cumbersome that Thomson's son, John, had to wheel them into the Assembly chamber. America's homeopathic profession was hardly strong enough to have played more than a subsidiary role in the struggle against licensure in New York, or any other state.[19]

It was not the repeal of the licensure laws that led to the formation of the A.M.A.; it was the conditions which led to repeal of those laws. The doctors sought to regain lost prestige by organizing to improve medical education. At the first "National Medical Convention," in 1846, there was no mention of homeopathy or sectarianism. The emphasis was clearly upon medical education and medical ethics.[20] During the second convention, in 1847, the committee on medical education reported that six reforms were absolutely necessary. These included the lengthening of the term of study from four to six months, and the institution of a three-year course (including two years as apprentice to a preceptor, and two six-month courses of lectures). The fourth recommendation was the only one that could have effected homeopathy. It stated that no college should accept a certificate of preparation from a preceptor who was "avowedly and notoriously an irregular practitioner."[21] That suggestion was clearly minor as compared with the major recommendations which preceded it.

In fact, the refusal to accept certificates from irregulars was hardly a hindrance to the development of homeopathy. It was simply too easy to establish homeopathic medical colleges which *would* accept certificates from irregulars. Furthermore, even the code of ethics should not be considered an attempt to throttle homeopathy. The introduction to the code, found in the *Proceedings of the Second National Medical Convention*, stated that the profession had no power to prevent, "or always to arrest" delusions. It could, however, "refuse to extend to them the slightest countenance, still less support." The consultation clause was not expected to seal the lid on the coffin of homeopathy. Rather, it was to prevent the orthodox profession from giving "support" to the homeopathic "quacks."[22]

If the Association had been formed to suppress homeopathy, the founders would not have waited six years to take the first real steps against it. The fact remains that not until 1852 and 1853 did the delegates become involved in serious discussion concerning their relations with sectarians.

[19] Kett, *Formation of the Profession*, pp. 20–21; Alexander Wilder, *History of Medicine* (New Sharon, Maine, 1901), pp. 503–10.
[20] *Proceedings of the National Medical Conventions*, pp. 15–22.
[21] Ibid., pp. 73–74.
[22] Ibid., p. 87.

It is true that the consultation clause forbade all intercourse with irregulars, but it is also true that not until 1855 did the A.M.A. demand that all state and local societies adopt the code of ethics.[23] If the threat from homeopathy had motivated the birth of the A.M.A., decisive action would have come earlier than 1855. Not until the 1870's did the A.M.A. insist that all member societies purge homeopaths from their ranks.

Rather interestingly, the American Institute of Homeopathy was founded for many of the same reasons as its orthodox counterpart, the American Medical Association. In July of 1843, the New York Homeopathic Physicians' Society invited interested homeopaths to a convention in New York. They convened at the Lyceum of Natural History on April 10, 1844. At that meeting, the Institute was established, with the stated purposes being: "Reformation and augmentation of the Materia Medica," and the "restraining of Physicians from pretending to be competent to practice Homeopathy who have not studied it in a skilful manner." The major problem troubling the homeopathic profession was that "the state of public information respecting the principles and practice of Homeopathy" was so defective that it was easy "for mere pretenders" to pass themselves off as qualified practitioners.[24] The "pretenders" who were able to take advantage of the increasing popularity of homeopathy were discrediting the homeopathic profession by their malpractices. As noted earlier, the orthodox physicians responded to a similar problem. To the allopaths, the difficulty was that poorly educated, almost illiterate men were being graduated annually from the medical schools. It would appear that rather than being formed to assault the other association, the two societies were established to reform the practice of medicine.

Another motive for the establishment of the American Institute of Homeopathy was the desire to scientifically investigate drug action. If truly objective experiments were carried out, the homeopaths hoped that the orthodox school would no longer "deride and oppose the contributions to the materia medica that have been made by the Homeopathic School."[25] Significantly, some allopaths also hoped that their society would become a truly scientific medical association, providing discussion of matters of

---

[23] *Transactions of the A.M.A.* 8 (1855): 56. From 1847 to 1852, a number of state and local societies purged themselves of homeopaths, largely in response to the A.M.A. code of ethics, but that action was not demanded by the A.M.A. For a scholarly study with a differing interpretation of this problem, see Harris L. Coulter, "Medicine and Public Opinion in the 19th Century United States," Ph.D. dissertation, Columbia University, 1969.

[24] *Transactions of the American Institute of Homeopathy* 1 (1846): 3.

[25] Ibid.

medical interest and a forum for innovations which would improve the practice of medicine.

If the popularity of the homeopaths had not been steadily increasing, it is conceivable that the orthodox profession might not have organized until many years later. On the other hand, the increasing respectability of homeopathy was indicative of the public disapproval of the allopaths. Worthington Hooker and Nathan Smith Davis, among others, recognized that the popularity of homeopathy was related to the inability of the orthdox school to keep its own house in order.[26] The A.M.A., then, was not formed to destroy homeopathy. It was established to raise the level of the medical practitioner so that the profession would regain its lost prestige and influence. Conversely, it was founded to improve orthodox medicine so that irregulars would no longer be able to attract patients.

The delegates to the 1853 A.M.A. convention discussed the relations between the regular profession and the homeopaths. On May 4 Dr. Edmund R. Peaslee, a professor at the Dartmouth Medical College and a pioneer in abdominal and pelvic surgery, rose to offer a resolution. The colleges, he declared, must refuse to examine students who intended to practice as irregulars. The following day Dr. P. Claiborne Gooch, a leading Virginia physician and a former editor of *The Stethoscope*, proposed that the colleges "administer to their graduates" a pledge that they would maintain "the honour and dignity of the profession; and that they will forfeit their degrees, whenever they desert the orthodox system of medicine." He also recommended that the colleges not graduate anyone who had not read and publicly sworn to abide by the code of ethics.[27] Although the pledge was never adopted, some schools did take the idea seriously. In 1860, for instance, a medical college in Savannah was reported to have made its graduates swear that they "will neither countenance nor affiliate with any system of irregular practice, nor engage either in the manufacture, sale, or recommendation of 'quack' nostrums or patent medicines, *nor countenance the practice of the senseless dogma of hydropathy, homeopathy, or Thompsonianism* [sic]" under penalty of revocation of diploma.[28]

The consultation clause of the code of ethics provided the profession with instructions for dealing with irregulars, although relatively ineffective ones. As an exclusive allopathic society, the A.M.A. did not need to enforce this section of the code. Some of its member societies, however, were not

---

[26] Hooker, *Physician and Patient*, passim; Davis, *History of the A.M.A.*, passim.
[27] *Transactions of the A.M.A.* 6 (1853): 40, 43–49.
[28] *North American Journal of Homeopathy* 9 (August 1860): 160.

chartered as strictly orthodox associations, and they began to take action. On February 6, 1850, the Massachusetts Medical Society accused Dr. Ira Barrows, of Norton, of dishonorable conduct, "for being the maker and vender at sundry different times of certain and several quack medicines," and "for being an irregular practitioner, having adopted the Homeopathic or Infinitesimal or Loaf sugar system." Since the charter of the Society provided for the membership of all qualified practitioners of good moral character, Barrows could not be denied fellowship simply because of his homeopathic tendencies. He had to be accused of other crimes. According to homeopathic sources, although other complaints were made against the doctor to ensure his expulsion, Barrows's crime was his practice of homeopathy.[29]

Events later in the same year, 1850, indicate that practicing homeopathy was not an offense punishable by expulsion. At the May 30 meeting of the Society, it was announced that a Salem doctor, Isaac Colby, had been converted to homeopathy, and that he had petitioned to resign his membership. He wrote that since he had renounced allopathic medicine, the fellows of the Society "felt themselves required to with-hold from me professional intercourse." Colby could not remain a member while his colleagues would not even speak to him. Three notable members of the Harvard Medical faculty, Dr. Oliver Wendell Holmes, Dr. J. B. S. Jackson, a pioneer pathologist and anatomist, and Dr. George Hayward, who in 1846 had performed the first major surgery under anesthesia, were appointed to decide whether the resignation should be accepted by the Society. Rather than simply debating Colby's resignation, the doctors became involved in a discussion as to whether homeopaths were qualified for fellowship in the Society. The committee believed that a homeopath who condemned the orthodox practices should certainly be expelled. They recognized, however, that many homeopaths sincerely believed in their system and were not ridiculing the actions of their allopathic colleagues. The committee debated whether they should be expelled along with their more vitriolic brothers.[30]

In their report to the Society, the committee admitted that homeopathy had, "at least indirectly, been of some service to the cause of medical

[29] Walter L. Burrage, *History of the Massachusetts Medical Society* (n.p., 1923), p. 97; *Publications of the Massachusetts Homeopathic Medical Society, 1840–1861* (Taunton, 1871), pp. 81–84.

[30] *Report of a Committee of the Massachusetts Medical Society on Homeopathy* (n.p., 1850), pp. 1–4; *Publications of the Massachusetts Homeopathic Medical Society*, p. 17.

science. It may have taught us," they declared, "to place more confidence in the curative powers of nature, and less in medicinal agents." After much soul-searching, they finally decided that a homeopath could resign, provided that he pay his back dues. They also recommended that diplomas from homeopathic colleges should no longer be accepted as evidence of a proper medical education.[31] The homeopathic colleges were certainly inferior to the leading orthodox schools, but they were probably no worse than the average ones. The Society was ensuring that future graduates of the homeopathic colleges would not automatically be admitted to fellowship. This practice was unfair in a day and age when graduates of regular schools who had received no more than a rudimentary medical education were accepted on the basis of their credentials. In view of the state of medical education, the Society would have done better if it had refused to accept any diplomas and instead had relied upon the recommendation of members and the results of examinations.

Other medical societies were confronted with the same problem, that of dealing with their homeopathic members. The Connecticut Medical Society, for instance, appointed a committee to decide whether local societies could expel three physicians reported to be "notoriously" practicing homeopathy. Dr. Worthington Hooker, the winner of the Fiske prize for the best essay denouncing homeopathy, was made chairman of the committee, which sealed the fate of the three homeopaths. In 1852 Hooker submitted his report, entitled: *The Treatment due from the Medical Profession to Physicians who become Homeopathic Practitioners.*[32] He asserted that the legislature had established the state medical society in order to guarantee "the services of a well-educated body of Physicians." The legislators presumed that "all medical opinions, and statements, and alleged discoveries, would be thoroughly examined and canvassed by the profession." The rise of medical sects in the past few years, he continued, had been an outgrowth of the development of radicalism in many aspects of American life. Since the advocates of each system had declared war against allopathic medicine, they had exiled themselves from professional society. He claimed that rather than allowing the profession to test new theories, they were appealing to the patients. Thus, the homeopaths, Hooker said, cannot "accuse us of exclusiveness or persecution."[33]

[31] Ibid.

[32] Worthington Hooker, *The Treatment due from the Medical Profession to Physicians who become Homeopathic Practitioners* (Norwich, Connecticut, 1852).

[33] Ibid., pp. 5–7.

The Connecticut physician then delved into the question at hand. "It is a well-known fact, however much it may be disputed in certain quarters, that the great majority of Homeopathic practitioners are not only poorly educated and destitute of any proper credentials, but that they are guilty of practicing the grossest arts of quackery." To the historian, Hooker's statement is false. In 1852 the majority of the homeopaths were graduates of the orthodox medical schools. They were, therefore, as well-educated as the average allopaths. Moreover, the homeopaths were convinced, not without justification, that their practices were more firmly based upon scientific experimentation than were the constantly changing orthodox practices. In any case, Hooker concluded that since the homeopaths were uneducated quacks, "any act of association with the common herd of Homeopathic practitioners should therefore be treated as a misdemeanor." Since the homeopaths who wage a "war of radicalism against the profession, seek to throw down the barriers that guard it from the intrusion of ignorance and quackery, if any of them be found in our ranks," Hooker asserted, "it was necessary for the profession to expel them." [34]

Hooker noted that it was commonly argued that although most homeopaths had adopted their system "for pecuniary reasons alone," there were a few who were honest in their convictions. Those few, the argument continued, should not be summarily dismissed. He replied to this line of reasoning by declaring that even if such a distinction could be made, which he doubted, "an honest conviction in favor of so gross a delusion may be justly considered as proving a mental obliquity so great, as to disqualify for the proper performance of the duties of a Physician." [35]

Some justice can be seen in Hooker's arguments. The homeopaths had been trying to convince the legislature to allow them to form their own society. If there were two societies, one orthodox and one homeopathic, a harmful precedent would be established. The advocates of any new theory could demand their own association, which in effect meant that its adherents would benefit from advertising as members of the state society. One should also keep in mind that since the society had lost its licensure power, it had become a club of physicians. Such a group could establish its own requirements for admittance, as well as expel members not living up to its standards. Unfortunately, such reasoning resulted in men being denied fellowship because of their beliefs.

The Chicago Medical Society provides another example of the use of the

[34] Ibid., pp. 5–9.
[35] Ibid., pp. 10–11.

consultation clause. In 1851 the association out of which the Society was born was struggling with the problem of professional ethics. In that year, Dr. J. E. McGin used "very abusive and unprofessional language towards the president of the society." When he was ordered to appear before a committee, McGin replied that the "society might go to h___ll." Dr. N. S. Davis, in his "Brief History of Medical Societies in Chicago," concluded his description of the episode by noting: "The name of Dr. McGin was stricken from the list of members, but the society did not prosper."[36]

Managing to struggle through its formative years, the society eventually was a viable organization with regular meetings. A committee was appointed on August 1, 1854, to "inquire into the *truth* of the report, that Dr. D. A. Colton, was engaged in the Homeopathic System of Practice in medicine." By the next meeting, Colton had admitted that he was indeed a practicing homeopath. This information was so incriminating that a resolution was immediately adopted ordering the secretary of the society "to Erase his name from its books." By adopting homeopathy, Colton "thereby forfeited all rights and title to membership." The next year, 1855, the doctors of Chicago formally adopted the A.M.A. code of ethics as their own moral guardian.[37]

The physicians of New York City reacted differently to the threat of homeopathy. The allopathic profession sought to emphasize the distinction between orthodoxy and homeopathy by establishing the New York Academy of Medicine as the city's orthodox society. At a meeting of the "Regular Practitioners of Medicine," on December 12, 1846, it was determined to organize an "Academy of Medicine." The primary objective was "The separation of the regular from irregular practitioners."[38] On February 3, 1847, at an early meeting of the Academy, it was evident that the membership was already having trouble keeping homeopathy out of the organization. Dr. J. R. Shearman admitted that he had violated the rules by consulting with a homeopath, and he was dropped from the rolls. The next month similar allegations were brought against Dr. W. W. Minor, but those charges were dropped and in the next year Minor was elected to the vice presidency.[39]

[36] N. S. Davis, "Brief History of Medical Societies in Chicago," in Chicago Medical Society, minutes, pp. 4–5, MS in Chicago Historical Society.
[37] Chicago Medical Society, minutes, August 1, 1854; September 5, 1854; September 4, 1855.
[38] F. Campbell Stewart to John W. Francis, New York, December 15, 1846, in Francis Papers, New York Public Library; Philip Van Ingen, *The New York Academy of Medicine; Its First Hundred Years* (New York, 1949), pp. 5–7.
[39] Ibid., pp. 15, 18.

New York's orthodox medical profession was not united behind the Academy. Dr. Edward H. Dixon, editor of the satirical medical journal, *The Scalpel*, maintained a running feud with the New York Academy of Medicine. In one editorial, he asserted that if the Academy was sincerely interested in the public welfare, it would not restrict membership to regular practitioners. The irregulars would profit from fellowship with such men of science, he said, and perhaps they might be shown their errors. Further, the "preservation of his patient's health" must remain the primary objective of all consultations, regardless of the practices of the consulting physicians. "If any one becomes *sincerely convinced*" that homeopathy is the best method of cure, "by all means adopt" it; "if not, in Heaven's name let their professors pass, with the ordinary interchange of gentlemanly courtesy, at least." Dixon insisted that the legitimate duty of the Academy was neither "to put down Homeopathy," nor to "stop advertising." Instead, he said, the Academy should do everything in its power to "improve in science, and to instruct the public how to preserve their health." [40] In calling for public health education, Dixon was almost a century ahead of his time. As late as the 1930's, the New York medical profession still had not reconciled itself to that need. In 1930, in fact, Health Commissioner Shirley Wynne resigned from the local medical societies when he was about to be expelled for the terrible crime of having advocated public health clinics. [41]

In summary, although not organized for that purpose, the American Medical Association set the stage for a concerted attack upon homeopathy. The code of ethics included a passage denying fellowship and forbidding consultation with irregular practitioners, and by the early 1850's, the orthodox societies were beginning to enforce the code. The orthodox profession had no means to destroy homeopathy, but by a strict enforcement of the consultation clause it was hoped that at least the new system would not benefit from assistance by the allopathic fraternity. By 1855, when the member societies of the A.M.A. had adopted the code of ethics, the battle lines were drawn between allopath and homeopath. The growth of the A.M.A. did not signal the end of homeopathy, but rather the polarization of the medical profession. The major effect of the birth of the American Medical Association upon homeopathy was that it was increasingly more difficult for an allopath to adopt homeopathy and remain a member of an

[40] *The Scalpel* 1 (January 1849): 40–42.
[41] See the *New York Times*, October 4, 1930, p. 19, col. 1; October 18, 1930, p. 16, col. 8; November 21, 1930, p. 20, col. 2.

orthodox society. In addition, of course, the allopathic profession possessed a national organization which would be necessary for an assault upon the "orthodox quackery" noted by Hooker, as well as homeopathy, the "unorthodox quackery."

V

THE DEMAND FOR "EQUAL RIGHTS"

THE MID-NINETEENTH CENTURY drive to establish municipal hospitals for the poorer segments of American society set the stage for an early confrontation between homeopathy and the orthodox medical profession. The continuing influx of immigrants was transforming America's quaint little towns into teeming cities reminiscent of England's industrial centers. The humanitarian movement from 1830 to 1860, which included abolition, temperance, woman's rights, and educational reform, also involved the construction of hospitals to care for the ills of the burgeoning population.

Medical care for the urban masses was almost nonexistent. Although some conscientious doctors offered free treatment to the poor, this approach left much to be desired. There were simply too many needy citizens and too few humanitarian physicians. In most cities there were several hospitals, which were commonly viewed as places where the poor went to die. The existing facilities, however, were insufficient to provide adequate medical care for the rapidly increasing population. In order to remedy the situation, city after city began to construct municipal hospitals.

As those institutions were being built, the homeopaths demanded their "right" to a number of wards. They argued that patients who were accustomed to homeopathic treatment should not be forced by their economic condition to undergo the "tortures" of heroic medicine. The first major battle between homeopathy and orthodoxy was to take place in Chicago, over control of the wards of the new municipal hospital. At the April, 1854, meeting of the Chicago Board of Health, city physician Brock McVickar was instructed to study the feasibility of establishing a hospital "commensurate with the actual wants and population of the city." He reported that a large institution was an absolute necessity. By 1857, after the completion of a series of conferences and studies, construction on the Chicago City Hospital was well under way.[1]

Chicago's homeopaths were in the midst of a severe financial crisis, possibly resulting from the depression of 1857. They were forced to close the doors of their hospital after only twenty-eight months of operation. The disciples of Hahnemann requested permission to treat homeopathically in the wards of the new hospital. On July 2, the Board of Health committee on hospitals replied to their petition, establishing two distinct medical staffs, one allopathic and the other homeopathic. Furthermore, it recommended that the patients be allowed to select their own "mode of treatment." Those with no preference would be shuffled back and forth between the two departments, going one week to the allopathic ward, the next week to the homeopathic. According to the plan, which would have paralyzed medical care of long-term cases, 25 per cent of the wards would be allocated to the homeopaths.[2]

Orthodox physicians were outraged at the Common Council for having adopted a course contrary to the A.M.A. code of ethics. How, they asked, could intelligent men allow "quacks" to treat their patients at the City Hospital? In July of 1857 the Chicago Medical Society passed a resolution forbidding its members to accept positions in "any hospital in part under the controll [sic] of irregular practitioners."[3] As a result of the apparently unexpected action of the allopaths, the Common Council hesitated to put its plan into operation. If the hospital were opened, the orthodox physicians would initiate a boycott. In that case the hospital would become strictly homeopathic. The city fathers were understandably reluctant to grant complete control to the minority group, especially since the orthodox profession included the city's most highly respected physicians.

The Common Council decided that it was better to take no action than to become embroiled in a complex medical dispute. As a consequence, the hospital was "unprovided" with furniture and supplies. In 1858, after a year of wrangling, the situation finally was resolved. The orthodox physicians leased the building and agreed to admit each resident at a cost to the

[1] *Report of the Board of Health of the City of Chicago for 1867, 1868 and 1869, and a Sanitary History of Chicago from 1833 to 1870* (Chicago, 1871), pp. 35–36, 43.

[2] Ibid., p. 46; Madge E. Pickard and R. Carlyle Buley, *The Midwest Pioneer; His Ills, Cures, and Doctors* (Crawfordsville, Indiana: 1945), pp. 215–16.

[3] Chicago Medical Society, minutes, July, 1857, MS in Chicago Historical Society.

city of three dollars per week.[4] Hostilities between allopath and homeopath ended with the homeopaths being denied access to the City Hospital and the city losing control of its own institution. Rather than being administered by a municipally appointed bureau, the hospital was operated by the orthodox medical profession, and for a time Chicago's poor were deprived of hospital care. Construction had been completed, but the doors remained locked until the hospital was leased by the allopaths. Only then, after a year of delay, could Chicago boast of a municipal hospital for its masses, but one under a different administration than originally planned.

In 1856, while the situation in the windy city was yet unresolved, the scene of battle shifted to New York. Early in the spring of that year, the Eleventh Street Homeopathic Dispensary asked the board of governors of the alms-house department to place some of the Bellevue wards under homeopathic control. A petition from New York's homeopathic physicians and their patients urged the board to accede to the request. Many prominent New Yorkers were among the thousands who signed the petition. These included, for example, Horace Greeley, the editor of the *New York Tribune*, and Charles Dana, the transcendentalist who was later to become editor of the *New York Sun*.[5] The homeopaths won the support of Benjamin F. Pinckney, a member of the board of governors, who introduced a resolution to place one-half of the wards under homeopathic control. Rather than make a rash decision, the board turned the question over to a three-man committee, consisting of Pinckney, Washington Smith, and P. G. Moloney.

The majority, Smith and Moloney, submitted a report opposed to the introduction of the new system. Over the past ten years, they declared, Bellevue had improved immeasurably. "From a lazar house to which the paupers even went with reluctance, it has become a well appointed Hospital, whose wards are crowded with grateful patients, and whose gates are thronged with eager applicants."[6] The two men noted that homeopathy was based upon a "wild transcendental theory." If that were not enough to condemn it, they asserted that homeopathy had been tested in Europe and found to be sadly lacking.

[4] *Report of the Board of Health*, p. 46; Bessie L. Pierce, *A History of Chicago* (New York, 1940), II, 449–50.

[5] *North American Homeopathic Journal* 6 (November 1857): 275.

[6] New York City. Department of Public Charities. Committee of the Board of Governors of the Alms House Department, *Majority and Minority Reports of the Select Committee of the Board of Governors, to whom was referred the subject of introducing Homeopathy into Bellevue Hospital, Submitted January 19, 1858* (Brooklyn, 1858), p. 4.

Smith and Moloney were familiar with *Homeopathy, and its Kindred Delusions*, the classic by Dr. Oliver Wendell Holmes. Repeating several of his arguments almost verbatim, they condemned the new system of medical practice. They compared homeopathy, for instance, to such "quackery" as the Perkins tractor. Again like Holmes, they acknowledged that homeopathy was widespread, but, they noted, so was every other "system of medical empiricism." The petitions favoring homeopathy came, the report continued, neither from the "inmates" of the hospital, who were to become the subjects of medical experimentation, nor from the "honest laboring classes of our city, whom the vicissitudes of life and the misfortunes of poverty may at any moment remove to the wards of Bellevue." Rather, they came from the homeopaths themselves and from a host of their wealthy clients, men who never would allow themselves to be taken to Bellevue.[7]

Smith and Moloney examined statistics of the European investigation of homeopathy, again borrowed from the Holmes essay. They noted, for instance, that in 1829 the King of Naples had established a commission to examine the new system. The result was a declaration that homeopathy had no effect other than preventing the employment of beneficial remedies. Five years later, in 1834, Andral, the French allopath, made a study of 140 cases in the Hospital de la Pitié and declared homeopathy to be a delusion. The majority report asked why the sick poor of New York were to be made the "subjects of an experiment" by a system which had "so repeatedly failed when put to the test of rigid investigation. If the curiosity of the few must be gratified," it continued, "why not choose the criminal for the experiment."[8]

Benjamin F. Pinckney submitted a minority report favoring the introduction of homeopathy. The new system, he said, was no longer an experiment; statistics from European and American hospitals demonstrate that years of investigation had proved the superiority of homeopathic medicine. Moreover, the new system was less expensive than the orthodox practices. Pinckney noted that the majority report was filled with inaccuracies. For instance, while the Naples study had denounced homeopathy, Pinckney asserted that two of the investigators had been so impressed with the potential of homeopathic medicine that they were converted to the newer system. In addition, a state paper was published criticizing the committee for

---

[7] Ibid., p. 9.

[8] Ibid.; see also *American Medical Times* (New York) 4 (January 18, 1862): 42–44.

having reported their prejudices rather than their findings. Pinckney declared that the Andral study suffered from a similar bias against homeopathy. The author of the minority report concluded by stating that since the cheaper and more effective system was employed by a significant percentage of the citizens of New York, the board of governors should let the homeopaths control some Bellevue wards.[9] After studying the two reports, however, the governors decided to let well enough alone. As in Chicago, New York's homeopaths were denied access to the wards of the municipal hospital.

In 1863 the scene of battle shifted once more, this time to Boston. Boston City Hospital, the object of great municipal pride, was scheduled to open its doors in May of 1864. The homeopathic profession demanded the "right" to treat their patients in the tax-supported institution. Albert J. Bellows, the leading spokesman for the new school of medical practice, petitioned the trustees of the "Free City Hospital." In his petition Bellows demonstrated, at least to his own satisfaction, that homeopathy was far superior to orthodox medicine. Moreover, the "scientific" methods of the new school prevented all the suffering from "lancets, hot irons, caustics, cataplasms, emetics, cathartics, and the whole paraphernalia of torments which so terrify patients and so disgrace the profession." Apart from protecting the patient from allopathic overdoses, and perhaps more important to the trustees, the tiny doses of homeopathy were less expensive than heroic medicines. Bellows then argued, with some justification, that it was cowardly and unfair to refuse to allow the homeopaths to admit their patients simply because the allopaths threatened a boycott. In "democratic America," the author declared, men were being denied their equal rights.[10]

After considering the evidence, the trustees finally ruled that the scheme to introduce homeopathy was impractical. It would, they said, "be fatal to the harmony necessary to the full success and usefulness of the new hospital."[11] Thomas C. Amory, Jr., the alderman who was president of the hospital's board of trustees, noted that the homeopaths had flocked to his office demanding admission to the medical staff. Such "radical differences of professional opinion exist between their practitioners and the regular faculty," he said, "that any attempt to combine both methods of cure under

[9] *North American Journal of Homeopathy* 6 (May 1858): 433–57.

[10] Albert J. Bellows, *A memorial to the Trustees of the Free City Hospital, with Statistics and facts, showing the comparative merits of Homeopathy and Allopathy, as shown by Treatment in European Hospitals* (Boston, 1863), pp. 23–25.

[11] *Report on the Introduction of Homeopathy into the City Hospital* (Boston, 1864), pp. 1–6.

the same roof, must inevitably lead to contention." Amory asserted that the allopathic medical board was fully competent to investigate the new systems and to integrate the best of them into the orthodox practices at the hospital. In any case, he argued, in order to maintain harmony it would be better for the city to endow a separate homeopathic hospital.[12]

As will be seen in a later chapter, during the 1880's homeopaths began to gain admittance to the wards of the various municipal hospitals. During the earlier period, however, from 1850 to 1880, the orthodox practitioners refused to serve alongside homeopaths in any hospital, and their opposition to homeopathy prevented the integration of the medical boards. In 1873, for instance, the board of managers of Pennsylvania's Harrisburg Hospital elected a regular medical staff. Dissension arose when several homeopaths offered to treat gratuitously if the hospital provided them with homeopathic medicines. When the board voted to accept the offer, two of its members, Drs. Curwen and Reily, resigned, and the entire allopathic staff followed their example. They could not remain affiliated with a hospital, they declared, which included a practice "so utterly at variance with that in which we have been educated." On August 7 the Dauphin County Medical Society announced its endorsement of "the manly and high-toned professional action" of the medical staff.[13]

The confrontation between orthodox medicine and its most powerful foe was not restricted to the personnel problems of the emerging hospitals. Every development which involved the employment of physicians provided a new battlefield in the struggle. The scene was set for another clash, for instance, when the shelling of Fort Sumter signalled the beginning of America's bloody Civil War. The large numbers of casualties from the early battles indicated that additional hospitals and many more surgeons were needed. In January of 1862 the homeopaths began to demand "equal footing in the army with any other medical school." The Army Military Board decided almost immediately that the admittance of homeopaths would be an invitation to "all schools of 'quack doctors.'"[14] For that reason, homeopaths were denied the privileges given orthodox physicians, and the

---

[12] City of Boston, Document number 40, *Proceedings at the Dedication of the City Hospital, May 24, 1864* (Boston, 1864), p. 42.

[13] *Medical and Surgical Reporter* (Philadelphia) 29 (August 23, 1873): 143; *Hahnemannian Monthly* 9 (September 1873): 92–94.

[14] *New York Times*, January 11, 1862, p. 4; for a complete examination of the process of appointing surgeons, see George W. Adams, "Health and Medicine in the Union Army, 1861–1865" (unpublished Ph.D. dissertation, Harvard University, 1946), pp. 14–20.

wounded were denied the advantages of homeopathy over the heroic practices.

Refusing to admit defeat, the homeopaths brought the issue into the halls of Congress. Senator James W. Grimes, a homeopathic supporter from Iowa, introduced a bill "to increase the efficiency of the medical department of the army." Senate bill 188, which appeared to be above politics, would have given the President the right to make enough appointments to expand and improve the medical department of the army. The bill was deceptive, however, as the new appointees were to come from either the regular army corps or from the "volunteer" surgeons. In effect, then, the President would be given the power to appoint anyone, even homeopaths. Oregon's Senator James W. Nesmith vigorously opposed the bill on the grounds that it would transform positions in the medical corps into choice political plums. He declared: "I guaranty that if Esculapius or Galen, said to be the fathers and founders of the medical science, were this day living, and were to come here themselves and make application, they could not get sufficient political influence to obtain these appointments." [15]

Nesmith swept aside the claim that the bill was necessary in order to give the troops a choice of physicians. How many doctors would be needed, he asked, if each and every soldier demanded the services of his family physician? The Senator noted that the committee on military affairs had heard from a number of medical sects, each demanding the "right" to be included in the medical corps. "The other day there was a spiritualist who desired to come before the committee, in order to organize a corps of spiritual rappers to draw wagons out of the mud." There were so many spiritualists in the army, that petitioner had declared, that there ought to be a medical corps of "mediums." After being briefly interrupted by a Senator who facetiously suggested that if nothing else would get the wagons out of the mud, perhaps rapping might be tried, Nesmith continued with his remarks. It was insane, he said, to "introduce clairvoyancers, spiritual rappers, homeopathists" and other medical sectarians, simply in order "to gratify the caprice of every soldier who happens to be in the army." [16]

Henry Wilson, the radical Republican senator from Massachusetts, who later was to write a *History of the Rise and Fall of the Slave Power in America*, noted that the old school allopaths had a stranglehold upon the medical boards that examined applicants for medical commissions. The

[15] *Congressional Globe*, 37 Cong.; 2 sess. (1862), p. 987.
[16] Ibid., p. 996.

orthodox physicians simply rejected all irregular practitioners. Although his early remarks seemed to favor the introduction of homeopathy, Wilson went on to state that sectarianism would lead to "great confusion" in diagnosis and treatment.[17] After more debate than the bill seemed to warrant, it passed both houses and was signed into law by President Lincoln.

The orthodox medical societies rushed into session to protest against the impending introduction of homeopathy into the medical corps. In fact, before the bill had even been passed, the New York Academy of Medicine passed a resolution prepared by one of New York's leading physicians, Dr. Valentine Mott. After years of testing, homeopathy had failed to establish itself in Europe, the resolution declared. Furthermore, the old world was familiar with homeopathy, and it still did not allow it into the military. The Academy asserted that homeopathy was "no more worthy" of introduction into the service than "kindred methods of practice as closely allied to quackery." Finally, Mott argued that the reduction of standards necessary to admit homeopathy would demoralize the entire medical corps.[18]

The orthodox profession actually had little to fear. Grimes's bill did not flood the military with homeopathic surgeons. The reason for the continued lack of homeopathic surgeons was simply that Presidential approval was necessary for appointment. The emancipator of the Negro slave was yet unwilling to unlock the doors for the medical heretic.[19]

The homeopaths were more frustrated than ever. Angered over their inability to enlist in the medical corps, the members of the Massachusetts Homeopathic Medical Society demanded that Congress immediately enlist homeopathic surgeons. The Society declared in a petition, that despite evidence that homeopathy was superior to allopathic medicine, the Medical Commission of Massachusetts had voted to reject all homeopathic applicants. Moreover, the army medical board, located in the nation's capital, "has sedulously endeavored to exclude from the Army all homeopathic surgeons, and from the army hospitals all homeopathic practice." The resolution insisted that a homeopathic surgeon be appointed whenever a "considerable portion" of the officers and men in a brigade requested one. In addition, army hospitals should provide for the homeopathic treatment of those who desire it. Finally, since allopaths cannot "intelligently" ex-

[17] Ibid., p. 997.
[18] Boston Medical and Surgical Journal 66 (February 6, 1862): 33–34; Philip Van Ingen, The New York Academy of Medicine: Its First Hundred Years (New York, 1949), p. 119.
[19] Milton Shute, Lincoln and the Doctors (New York, 1933), p. 94, cited in Adams, "Health and Medicine," pp. 126–28.

amine homeopaths in their specialty, the Society urged the creation of a separate examining board to pass upon the qualifications of homeopathic applicants.[20]

Homeopathic journals became filled with articles which condemned the homeopathic exclusion from the military. John T. Temple, a professor at the Homeopathic Medical College of Missouri, was author of one of the more unforgettable of these. In an article entitled "Humanity, Homeopathy, and the War," Temple asked whether the best surgeons had been selected to minister to the Union's valiant defenders. Eloquently he replied: "The sad hearts of widowed thousands exclaim, no! Thousands of mothers bereft of their sons by ignorant and incompetent physicians cry: No! No!" Homeopathy, he said, would save the lives of the thousands who were being overdosed with allopathic medicines. The American soldier, he asserted, had the right to select his own physician, especially since his life was at stake in the process. Moreover, homeopathy would not only provide improved medical care but also a less expensive method of treatment.[21]

A St. Louis homeopath, Dr. E. C. Franklin, described his experiences as an army surgeon. When there was a lack of trained physicians in the west, he was appointed surgeon to the 5th Regiment, Missouri Volunteers. After weathering an attack upon his qualifications by the allopathic profession, Franklin assumed his position. Assigned to the hospital at Mound City, near Cairo, Illinois, he used homeopathic remedies upon those who were considered "beyond recovery." Franklin claimed that with the assistance of two others, Drs. Pratt and Wales, homeopathy had restored 30 per cent of those men to good health. After hearing a number of vociferous complaints about the "quacks" in the army, H. R. Wirtz, the medical director of the Department of the Tennessee, ordered an investigation. Pratt was soon forced to resign, and despite his successes, Franklin was relieved of his duties.[22]

Although insistent in their demands, the homeopaths were prevented from joining their allopathic colleagues at the bedside of the wounded. Orthodox control of the medical examining boards was too powerful, and the regular profession was able to prevent the medical heresy from slipping into the military. The fact that doctors were always in short supply was

[20] See *Boston Medical and Surgical Journal* 66 (March 20, 1862): 163.

[21] John T. Temple, "Humanity, Homeopathy, and the War," *North American Journal of Homeopathy* 11 (November 1862): 161–68.

[22] E. C. Franklin, "Homeopathy in the Army," *North American Journal of Homeopathy* 12 (November 1863): 267–78.

beside the point, and despite the fact that many homeopaths offered their services, the medical corps remained an allopathic bastion.

Ironically, at the time when the homeopaths were insisting that orthodoxy was only hurrying the wounded to early graves, Surgeon-General William A. Hammond issued his famous circular number six. Hammond's order of May 1863 forbade the issue of calomel and tartar emetic to the medical corps. This was an insult to the integrity of the profession, implying, correctly in some cases, that the allopaths were overdosing their patients. Furthermore, it inferred that physicians were incapable of selecting their treatments. In effect, the medical corps was being told that although they wanted to administer calomel and tartar emetic, the Surgeon-General would no longer allow them to poison their patients. Needless to say, though some orthodox physicians were pleased to see calomel banished from the medicine chest, circular number six provoked a storm of outraged indignation,[23] but although allopathic treatment left much to be desired, homeopathy was still denied access to the military.

The next major dispute between the schools of practice occurred in 1870. The United States Pensions Commissioner, Dr. H. Van Aernam, decided that uniformity was vital to the morale and operation of his department. He wrote to inform three homeopathic examining surgeons, Drs. Stillman Spooner, A. T. Bull, and Courtland Hoppin, of their dismissal. Van Aernam explained that "all Examining Surgeons for the Bureau should belong to one school, and adopt one theory of medicine."[24] The orthodox profession applauded the action of the Commissioner; the editor of the *Medical and Surgical Reporter*, for instance, asserting that it was important for the same criteria to be used in diagnosing and reporting ailments. "Notoriously, this were impossible," he continued, if homeopaths, eclectics, and all "the other riff-raff of irregular doctors," were appointed to the Pensions Bureau. True to its role as a crusading force against sectarianism, the New York Academy of Medicine also approved of Van Aernam's action.[25]

Representative James Garfield, the future President, entered the affair. He was a personal friend of several "radical" allopaths who openly con-

---

[23] This controversy is described by Gert H. Brieger, "Therapeutic Conflicts and the American Profession in the 1860's," *Bulletin of the History of Medicine* 41 (May–June 1967): 215–22; see also *Transactions of the A.M.A.* 14 (1863): 29–34, and the *Medical Communications of the Massachusetts Medical Society* 11 (Boston, 1874): 162.

[24] *New England Medical Gazette* 6(February 1871): 73–77.

[25] *Medical and Surgical Reporter* 24 (March 18, 1871): 216; Van Ingen, *New York Academy of Medicine*, p. 146.

sulted with any qualified physician, including Negroes, women, and homeopaths. Their actions, which will be detailed in a later chapter, brought the two "radicals," Drs. D. W. Bliss and C. C. Cox, into a close alliance with homeopathy. Garfield introduced a bill to secure "equal rights in the civil service of the United States for the medical profession." The resolution, which among other things would have prohibited the dismissal of homeopaths from the Pensions Bureau, was quietly tabled in committee.[26]

The homeopathic profession rose to protest the "high-handed" dismissal of the three physicians. On April 12, 1871, the Massachusetts Homeopathic Medical Society demanded that Van Aernam be "speedily removed from office." The Society claimed that in removing Spooner, Bull, and Hoppin, the Commissioner had "publicly avowed and promulgated the Anti-American, proscriptive and pernicious doctrine, that an individual is ineligible to office under the national government, unless a member of a particular sect."[27] In the face of the ground swell of professional indignation, Van Aernam resigned his position, the three homeopaths were reinstated, and General J. H. Baker, the next commissioner, was soon able to report that surgeons were appointed "without regard to theories or schools." Baker demonstrated his tolerance, or at least his political acumen, by appointing a few homeopaths.[28]

In May of 1871 an episode similar to the Van Aernam case occurred in Massachusetts. Brigadier General I. S. Burrill appointed a Boston homeopath, Dr. Henry P. Shattuck, as brigade surgeon in the Massachusetts militia. The state surgeon-general, Dr. William J. Dale, refused to commission the irregular. When homeopaths complained, the press began to inquire. Dale responded to the public interest in the case by ordering the state medical commission to examine Shattuck. When it appeared that Dale would reject Shattuck after making him undergo the formalities, the homeopath refused to appear before the commission. At that point, Dale recommended to Governor Claflin that the recalcitrant homeopath be rejected.

On August 30 the Massachusetts Homeopathic Medical Society discussed the situation. A committee of twenty-five was appointed to meet with the governor. Faced by such a large group, the governor presumably would recognize the significance of the problem. On September 19 Claflin heard

[26] *Congressional Globe*, 41 Cong., 3 sess. (1870–71), p. 1701. For a discussion of the Bliss-Cox affair, see chap. VI.

[27] *Publications of the Massachusetts Homeopathic Medical Society, 1871–1877* (Boston, 1878), pp. 16–19.

[28] U.S. Commissioner of Pensions, *Report, 1872* (Washington, D.C., 1872), p. 11; *Medical Union* (N.Y.) 1 (February 1873): 37–38

the homeopaths, but he asserted that he had so much respect for his good friend Dale that he accepted all of his recommendations. Moreover, the governor said that if Shattuck were appointed, several men with seniority would be outranked by a younger man with no prior military experience. The homeopaths were outraged at the arrogance of the governor, but they could do nothing to remedy the "grave injustice." Dr. I. T. Talbot, Boston's leading homeopath, persuaded his more hot-tempered colleagues that it would be self-defeating to openly condemn the politically powerful governor, or even to demand that he dismiss his personal friend.[29] In spite of a lot of discussion and even more publicity, homeopathy gained little from the Shattuck affair.

Having opposed the orthodox restrictions upon irregular practice from 1850 to 1871, the homeopaths had failed to advance their position. Their only victory, over the Pensions Commissioner, may have been more imagined than real. After struggling to unseat Van Aernam, only a few irregulars were appointed as pension surgeons, and the army medical corps remained completely closed to homeopaths. A few irregular practitioners did manage to gain entry by neglecting to mention that they were homeopaths, but they were dismissed as soon as the truth became known. During and after the Civil War, the orthodox profession maintained complete control over the boards which passed upon the qualifications of all applicants for commissions. During the war, however, public opinion could not be mobilized by the homeopaths. Even the newspapers which were often sympathetic towards homeopathy agreed with the allopaths that its admission to the military could be disastrous to the health of thousands of soldiers. The editor of the *New York Times*, for example, asserted that homeopathy would only confuse the war effort. With "contending schools there could neither be system, order, nor unity in the treatment of disease."[30] In addition, while the nation was shocked by the ravages of war, the complaints of the irregular physicians fell upon deaf ears. The people had more important things to worry about than the "injustices" of the army medical corps.

The homeopaths, then, failed to gain the "right" to treat their patients in the municipal hospitals, and they also failed in their efforts to join the Union medical corps. Their only victory, in the Pensions Bureau, was a

---

[29] *New England Medical Gazette* 6 (August 1871): 356–59; (September 1871): 410–19; (October–November 1871): 471–75; *Publications of the Massachusetts Homeopathic Medical Society, 1871–77* (Boston, 1878), pp. 34–40.

[30] *New York Times*, January 11, 1862, p. 4.

Pyrrhic one, as homeopaths continued to be denied positions in the government service. The earliest confrontations between homeopathy and orthodox medicine proved to be decisive defeats for the advocates of the new school of practice.

VI

ENFORCING THE
CONSULTATION CLAUSE

DURING THE PERIOD of Reconstruction that followed the Civil War, the orthodox medical profession continued to assault the bastions of homeopathy. Having lost their powers of licensure during the Jacksonian period, the allopaths were unable to destroy their competition at one blow. A strict enforcement of the A.M.A. code of ethics, however, by prohibiting contact between the two schools, could prevent further conversions to sectarianism. The consultation clause was not only a means of separating "quackery" from orthodoxy, but it also was a public expression of contempt. It implied that sectarians were incompetents who were totally unfit professional associates. In the late 1860's the allopathic profession renewed its enforcement of the code.

The first step was to charge several leading allopaths with violating the consultation clause. On October 5, 1867, Dr. Augustus K. Gardner, one of the founders of the New York Academy of Medicine, faced such an accusation. He admitted consulting with Dr. Edward G. Bartlett, but he asserted that Bartlett was not then practicing homeopathy. In a letter to the Academy's committee on ethics, Gardner sought to explain the circumstances. He said that Bartlett, a personal friend, was a regular graduate who had married into a homeopathic family. After spending some time in the west, practicing according to Hahnemann, Bartlett returned to New York. Shortly after his arrival, he asked Gardner to "deliver a patient with forceps." Believing that he was not violating professional ethics, Gardner consented to assist his friend in the delivery. Unable to convince his colleagues of his innocence, Gardner was unceremoniously expelled from the Academy he had helped to establish.[1]

Following the example of the Academy, several other societies suspended a few members for having violated the consultation clause of the A.M.A. code of ethics. The American Medical Association, however, not content with taking the lead in the war against homeopathy, took an equally firm stand on other controversial issues. In 1868 the Association refused to open its doors to well-qualified lady doctors.[2] Two years later, it turned its back upon delegates from racially integrated societies, and subsequently it tabled a resolution which would have ensured that no delegate be excluded on account of race or color. The *New York Times* asked in an editorial if prejudice was not being carried to the extreme when the nation's doctors decreed: "You shall not be allowed to prescribe a dose of medicine, or at least not in consultation with us, unless you can change the color of your skin from black to white."[3]

Having disposed of their Negro and their female colleagues, the orthodox physicians returned to their homeopathic enemies. At the 1870 A.M.A. convention, two prominent Boston gynecologists, Drs. John L. Sullivan and Horatio R. Storer, objected to the seating of delegates from the Massachusetts Medical Society. The society had continually violated the code of ethics, they declared, by having "tolerated" homeopathic members. The A.M.A. committee on ethics investigated the allegation and soon reported that the charge had been substantiated. The committee recommended that unless the society "purge itself of irregular practitioners," it should not be entitled to representation at national conventions. When the delegates adopted the committee report, the eyes of the profession were suddenly focussed upon the Massachusetts Medical Society.[4] If this society did not expel its homeopathic members, even its orthodox members would be excluded from the professionally respectable A.M.A.

The first response of the Society came at a meeting held only three weeks after the ultimatum had been issued. When it was proposed to force the

[1] New York Academy of Medicine, Committee of Ethics, Minutes, September 30, 1867, in MS scrapbook housed at the Academy. See also Van Ingen, *The New York Academy of Medicine: Its First Hundred Years* (New York, 1949), p. 141; *New York Times*, October 18, 1867, p. 4, col. 7.

[2] *Transactions of the A.M.A.* 19 (Philadelphia, 1868): 25, 28–29.

[3] Ibid. 21 (Philadelphia, 1870): passim; see commentary in *New York Times*, May 7, 1870, p. 6, col. 5; and the *Boston Evening Transcript*, May 7, 1870, p. 4, col. 2.

[4] *Transactions of the A.M.A.* 21 (Philadelphia, 1870): 29; Walter L. Burrage, *History of the Massachusetts Medical Society* (Boston, 1923), pp. 127–30.

district societies to expel all homeopaths, Dr. Holt, a homeopath from Lowell, tried to speak. He was "met with a storm of hisses." Removing his coat, he threw it upon the platform, declaring that he had the floor and would be heard even if he had to wait until the time for dinner had passed. Order could not be restored, and Holt was unable to explain his position. After the stormy confrontation, Dr. Sullivan offered a resolution to dismiss all doctors "who publicly profess to practice in accordance with any exclusive dogma, whether calling themselves homeopaths, hydropaths, eclectics, or what not, in violation of the Code of Ethics of the American Medical Association."[5] Proud of their action, convinced that they had satisfied the demands of the national convention, the members of the Society adjourned to their homes. The editor of the *Boston Medical and Surgical Journal*, however, insisted that the expulsion of homeopaths was illegal. He explained that the charter of the Society provided for the membership of every physician of good moral character, regardless of his system of practice.[6]

When they realized that their resolution meant very little, the councillors of the Society reconvened. A committee reported, interestingly, that Drs. Storer and Sullivan should be condemned for having made an accusation against the Society without first having informed the delegates. The charges presented by the two physicians were declared to be "an act of discourtesy which deserves censure." After having reprimanded Storer and Sullivan, the committee turned its wrath upon the A.M.A. The attempt to impose conditions upon the Society, it asserted, was "ill-conceived and unwarranted." Accepting the recommendations of the committee, the councillors unanimously voted to censure both Storer and Sullivan. They then decided to boycott national conventions until the A.M.A. reconsidered its action.[7]

Although the allopaths considered homeopathy to be no better than common "quackery," the Massachusetts Medical Society had not expelled its homeopathic members. The councillors recognized that expulsion might be illegal and that it would only further discredit the Society in the eyes of the press and the public. Instead of dismissing the homeopaths, the councillors had vented their rage upon Storer and Sullivan, whom they considered responsible for publicizing the situation. Similarly, the American Medical

[5] *Medical Communications of the Massachusetts Medical Society* 11 (Boston, 1874): appendix, pp. 158–59.

[6] *Boston Medical and Surgical Journal* 83 (July 28, 1870): 59–62; *Boston Morning Journal*, May 26, 1870, p. 1, col. 4.

[7] *Medical Communications of the Massachusetts Medical Society* 11, appendix, pp. 194–95.

Association was condemned for having been consistent in its opposition to homeopathy. The action of the councillors represented, then, an interesting turn of events.

On February 1, 1871, the councillors once again adopted a series of resolutions providing for the expulsion of any fellow who either joined a sectarian organization, or who practiced according to an "exclusive dogma or theory." Rather than preparing a bill of indictment against practicing homeopaths, the councillors followed that action by drafting a letter to the A.M.A. They explained that the Society was a public institution which could not expel members who were sectarians. In addition to the legal question, the councillors insisted that "more serious mischief will result to the profession and to medical science" by the attempt to remove homeopaths from the society, than by "quietly ignoring them." The letter went on to explain that the original resolution expelling irregulars could not be legally binding. It could "only be regarded as expressing the earnest wish of the Society to rid itself of the various classes of persons named in it."[8]

When it became apparent that the American Medical Association would not reconsider its position, the state society realized that firm action was necessary to ensure recognition of the Massachusetts profession. A resolution was adopted which provided that any fellow who enrolled in an organization based upon an "exclusive theory or dogma" did so in violation of the by-laws of the society.[9] As noted above, that resolution was hardly an unfamiliar one. The society had taken a similar step several times in the past, but it had never taken action to implement the resolution. In 1850 the society had examined its relationship with irregulars, and decided that homeopaths who paid their back dues could honorably resign. In 1859 the members had voted to expel "homeopaths, spiritualists, and Thomsonians." Discretion had seemed the better part of valor, however, and there were no dismissals.[10] Now, in 1871, the ultimatum of the A.M.A. forced the society to act against its homeopathic members. Eight physicians—Drs. William Bushnell, Milton Fuller, H.L.H. Hoffendahl, George Russell, Israel T. Talbot, David Thayer, Benjamin West, and William Gregg—were summoned to appear before a board of trial. Significantly, the society was reluctant to initiate proceedings against its homeopathic members. Expulsion was probably illegal, and, in any case, it would only benefit homeopathy by providing more martyrs to the cause.

[8] Ibid., pp. 201–9.
[9] *Boston Medical and Surgical Journal* 88 (February 20, 1873), pp. 197–98.
[10] I. T. Talbot, *The Common Sense of Homeopathy* (Boston, 1862), pp. 1–26.

Newspaper opinion was clearly on the side of the persecuted homeopaths. The *Boston Daily Journal* declared that "it seems pitiable that these men, nearly all of whom have been educated at Harvard University and pronounced thoroughly competent to practice medicine, and who have so long enjoyed the confidence and respect of the community, should be consigned to so fearful a doom." It was, the editor said, "a sad warning to those who believe in the 'freedom of public opinion.'"[11] A *Boston Evening Traveller* reporter noted that the homeopaths were willing to discuss professional matters with the press. They were "quite free from the prejudice of the 'regulars' against matters of ethics being known to the 'laity'."[12] The injustices of the trial would soon have the press even more firmly behind the homeopaths.

Newspapers did print a number of pertinent letters to the editor. One to the *Boston Journal*, for instance, agreed with the position of the medical society. The writer, who signed himself "A. R. B.," compared the situation to politics and religion. He asked rhetorically whether the Republican convention could be condemned for ejecting a Democrat, or whether a Unitarian convocation could be censured for refusing to seat a Catholic.[13] His argument, however, could only be employed in reference to organizations like the American Medical Association or the New York Academy of Medicine. The Massachusetts Medical Society, unlike the others, was neither chartered nor intended to be an exclusively allopathic fraternity. It was to include all competent and qualified practitioners, regardless of their medical theories.

In any case, on November 21, 1871, Boston became a battleground in the war between allopathy and homeopathy. At the beginning of the trial, Talbot, one of the accused, asked the Society to specify which "dogma and theory" he was charged with practicing. It was a maneuver to demonstrate that the homeopaths were being persecuted for the "crime" of being irregular practitioners, rather than for being immoral, injudicious, or unqualified. After a short conference, the word "homeopathic" was inserted in the formal indictment. Talbot then tried to read a protest. The chairman of the board of trial, Dr. George Hayward, dismissed it by saying, "We sha'n't pay any regard to that." David Thayer, one of the homeopaths on trial, then declared, "We'll find something you will pay attention to." At

---

[11] *Boston Daily Journal*, November 8, 1871, p. 2, col. 4. See also ibid., November 21, 1871, p. 4, col. 1.
[12] *Boston Evening Traveller*, November 21, 1871, p. 1, cols. 2–6.
[13] *Boston Journal*, November 20, 1871, p. 4, col. 1.

that point, John B. Dearborn, deputy sheriff of Suffolk County, marched into the hall with an injunction forbidding the society to expel any members. According to the report in the *Boston Journal*, the unexpected turn of events "made considerable of a commotion."[14] It shocked the physicians who had assembled to drum the heretics out of the society, and after some discussion, the proceedings were recessed while the doctors all awaited the results of a legal battle over the right of the society to expel members.

Since the status of the American medical profession was quite low and doctors were the butt of innumerable jokes, the editor of the *Boston Post* did not hesitate to publish a satirical account of the "war." The *Post* reporter described his reaction to the "battlefield." He could smell the "musty bandages" of the killed and wounded. He stood thunderstruck as he watched the "hosts of Homeopathy and Allopathy moving up," with "drawn scalpels," "terrible *tourniquets*," "murderous *ecraseurs*, amputating saws, and lancets glittering in the sunlight." He could only shudder as he awaited the collision of the opposing forces and the inevitable "casting of the leeches by phlegmatic grenadiers." Early in December the *Post* disappointedly announced to its readers that the battle had ended "without the loss of a man on either side." "There was no bombardment of boluses, no fusillade of medicated pellets, no valiant charge with amputating instruments. The attacking party withdrew before a gun was fired."[15]

While physicians on both sides were disturbed over the implications of the trial, and while the press was expressing either anger at the attack upon liberty or amusement at the sight of dignified physicians preparing for battle, patent medicine manufacturers were quick to take advantage of the situation. The *Boston Journal* of November 25 included an advertisement that declared, "It is a singular fact that while Allopaths and Homeopaths are fighting desperately over a principle that neither understand, and about which the public care nothing, invalides everywhere are rejoicing that in VEGETINE is found the 'elixer of life.'"[16]

Talbot, the leading homeopath under indictment, was elected president of the American Institute of Homeopathy. In his inaugural address of May 21, 1872, he proclaimed that "Boston, which tortured witches, banished Baptists, and hung Quakers," in 1871 "has found among its citi-

[14] *Boston Journal*, November 21, 1871 (evening ed.), p. 2, col. 3; p. 3, col. 5. A similar report is given in the *Boston Post*, November 22, 1871, p. 3, cols. 3–4.
[15] *Boston Post*, November 23, 1871, p. 3, cols. 3–4; December 6, 1871, p. 1, col. 8.
[16] *Boston Journal*, November 25, 1871, p. 4, col. 5.

zens some who, if not allowed to be wicked, are more foolish than any who had infested its streets two centuries before." Rather than destroying homeopathy, he declared that the zeal of the Massachusetts Medical Society had only won the condemnation of the press. Moreover, in the state of pro-homeopathic sentiment whipped up by the encounter, a fair opened to finance the struggling homeopathic hospital had raised over $100,000 in only two weeks.[17]

The following February, 1873, when the trustees of Boston University were about to establish a medical college, they looked to the martyred homeopaths to provide the faculty. The attack upon sectarianism played a role in attracting this windfall to the cause of homeopathic medicine. In addition, it was widely recognized that the accused were not at all incompetent. Among them were some of the most highly respected physicians in the community. Dr. Talbot, for instance, had a large practice and was the personal physician to many leading Bostonians, including Isaac Rich, a founder of the University.[18]

On February 15, two days after the homeopaths were asked to establish the medical department at Boston University, the state supreme court ruled that the society did, in fact, have the power of expulsion.[19] The society prepared to resume its trial of the eight homeopaths. Dr. Oliver Wendell Holmes, however, had second thoughts about continuing the proceedings. In a letter to Dr. John Collins Warren, Boston's leading surgeon and a founder of the Massachusetts General Hospital, Holmes suggested that the charges be dropped, "now that a point had been made." The homeopaths, he said, "would like a chance to answer an attack, and they would at once be lifted into notice by the article which was meant to finish them." He reminded Warren of the wisdom of two maxims: "let sleeping dogs lie," and "to let well enough alone." As long as public opinion considered the homeopaths "a wronged and persecuted band of martyrs," the profession, he said, could derive little benefit from their expulsion.[20]

It is interesting to note that Holmes's advice was totally inconsistent with his treatment of irregulars thirty years earlier. In his essay, *Homeopathy,*

---

[17] *Transactions of the American Institute of Homeopathy, 1872* (Philadelphia, 1872), p. 181.

[18] *Medical Investigator* (Chicago) 10 (June 1873): 380–81; *Hahnemannian Monthly* 9 (October 1873): 130; Frederick C. Waite, *History of the New England Female Medical College, 1848–1874* (Boston, 1950), p. 100.

[19] *New England Medical Gazette* 8 (March 1873): 129–30.

[20] Holmes to Warren, Boston, April 14, 1873, in Warren papers, Massachusetts Historical Society.

and Its Kindred Delusions, Holmes had insisted that medical "delusions" should be ruthlessly suppressed. Now, in 1871, he wanted to "let well enough alone." Besides being a change from his previous position, his recommendations could not have solved the problem at hand—the A.M.A. ultimatum. The delegates of that Association would be satisfied with nothing less than the banishment of all the homeopathic "quacks." If Holmes's advice were heeded, the society would have no representation at A.M.A. conventions and its members would continue to remain outside the national circle of respectable allopathic physicians.

Disregarding the warning of Dr. Holmes, on April 29, 1873, the Massachusetts Medical Society resumed the trial of homeopathy. A five-man board of trial was appointed, which consisted of Drs. Jeremiah Spofford of Groveland, Augustus Torrey of Beverley, George Hayward of Boston, Frederic Winsor of Winchester, and Francis C. Greene of Easthampton. One of the accused, Dr. Samuel Gregg, had died while the legal battle was being fought, and so there were only seven defendants. The homeopaths were charged with "Conduct unbecoming and unworthy an honorable physician and member of this Society." This "Conduct" was "practicing or professing to practice according to an exclusive theory or dogma, and belonging to a Society whose purpose is at variance with the principles of, and tends to disorganize the Massachusetts Medical Society." [21] The issue was clear; the defendants were charged with practicing homeopathy and with membership in the Massachusetts Homeopathic Medical Society.

Talbot, appearing as counsel for William Bushnell, began his defense. He declared that since the trial was a matter of public interest, the press should be admitted to the hall. The board ruled that it was a private matter; only members of the society could be present. That decision was clearly in line with professional thought. Publicity given to ethical violations would benefit neither the defendant nor the society. After his first request had been rejected, Talbot declared that the secretary had incorrectly transcribed the session of November 21, 1871 and that a "phonographic reporter" was required. That, like his first demand, was given short shrift.

---

[21] *Trial of William Bushnell, Samuel Gregg, George Russell, David Thayer, Milton Fuller, H. L. H. Hoffendahl, I. T. Talbot, Benjamin H. West, all of Boston, for practicing Homeopathy, while they were members of the Massachusetts Medical Society* (Boston, 1873), p. 4. This pamphlet is a verbatim copy of the Massachusetts Medical Society, Records of the Boards of Trial, 1858–1881, MS in possession of the Society, pp. 69–162. Newspaper accounts were provided by the homeopathic defenders, but testify to the accuracy of the Society's version. See, for instance, *Boston Evening Transcript*, April 29, 1873, p. 8, cols. 4–6; *Boston Globe*, April 30, 1873, p. 8, cols. 3–4; *Boston Post*, April 30, 1873, p. 4, cols. 1–2.

Next, the board rejected a request for legal counsel. Finally, the society refused to recess the trial in order to allow the preparation of a proper defense.[22]

When the society denied the defendants those basic legal rights, the press openly sympathized with the homeopaths. The *Boston Post* declared that "to those who have no medical theory to support, the protest and the answer of the accused members seem to be strongly sustained by considerations of equity and law." The trial, the editor said, was nothing more than an "inquisition." The defendants had been denied the right to challenge witnesses, the benefit of legal counsel, or even the power to exclude jurors who had previously declared against them. Moreover, since the board of trial was serving as prosecutor as well as jury, it made a mockery of the American legal system. In conclusion, the *Post* asserted that "in the attempt to expel members who follow their honest convictions, the fruit of study, experience and practice, in the treatment of disease, it will be difficult to convince unprejudiced men that an act of great illiberality is not contemplated."[23]

Dr. Benjamin West opened his defense immediately after Talbot's demands had been rejected by the board. West argued that the resolution passed by the society on June 7, 1871, was an *ex post facto* law, thus contrary to the United States Constitution. That resolution had provided that members who practiced homeopathy did so in violation of the by-laws. West claimed that it only could refer to physicians not yet admitted to fellowship. He said, moreover, that the resolution was contrary to the American Bill of Rights because it denied free thought and free speech. West went on to argue against the legality of the board of trial. He insisted that a board could not try or expel members. That power, he explained, was vested in the society as a whole. The precedent was set in 1836, when Dr. John S. Bartlett was tried before the entire society. West had cogently argued against the legality of the actions of the society, and he had thrown doubt upon the validity of the trial itself.

West then discussed the changing state of medical practice. He said that he learned in school that cupping and leeching were among the more beneficial treatments. Medicine, however, was as changeable as "the kaleidoscope." Was he to kill his patients with heroic medicines, or was he to "adopt the more modern and scientific method of treatment?" By expelling

[22] *Trial of William Bushnell*, p. 5.
[23] *Boston Post*, May 1, 1873, p. 1, col. 7.

homeopaths, the state society, he asserted, was "merely repeating the experiment of King Canute in forbidding the advance of the tide. It may succeed in removing their names from the catalogue, but," he asked, "will it have abolished the cause of difference?"[24] After West had completed his defense, the board of trial agreed to adjourn for a fortnight, ostensibly in order to allow time for the defense to be prepared, but possibly for the prosecution to discuss the points argued by Doctor West.

The climax of the proceedings came in two weeks, when Talbot eloquently rose in his own defense. After asserting that homeopathy was superior to orthodox medicine and denying that the homeopathic society was in any way opposed to the state society, Talbot demonstrated his mastery of nineteenth-century rhetoric. He declared that "all history shows that truth is helped by narrow and malignant attacks upon her. She gains more from the malice of her enemies than even from the ability of her friends." The physicians in the hall must have had misgivings about their actions when Talbot noted: "Already we have proof that coming generations will have reason to be thankful for the unsuccessful assault upon us last year. The cordial sympathy and world-wide notice it got us, poured into our hands the means to found and most liberally endow a Homeopathic Hospital to relieve the sufferings of future generations." The results of the Boston trial, he predicted, "will be to give us still larger and kinder support. A second wave of public sympathy will found a University for the study of our system. . . . If you, gentlemen, can afford to contribute thus lavishly to our success, we surely should not quarrel with the prominence and popularity you give us."[25]

Even Talbot's threat did not deter the members of the board; on May 19, 1873, they announced their decision. Of course, it must be understood that the trial was never intended to be unbiased. The board paid little attention to the oratory. The trial was a necessary formality in order to expel the homeopaths. The defendants were found guilty and ordered dismissed from the society. The membership soon voted to adopt the ruling of the board of trial, and the society had rid itself of sectarians. After 1873 the society continued to seek out the heretics in its midst. Two more homeopaths, Drs. Herbert C. Clapp and H. L. Chase, were dismissed on December 22, 1874. Two weeks later Dr. Floyd G. Kittredge, an orthodox practitioner, was expelled for being an abortionist, and in a "disgraceful state of

---

[24] *Boston Evening Transcript*, May 1, 1873, p. 2, col. 6; *Trial of William Bushnell*, pp. 40–51.
[25] *Trial of William Bushnell*, p. 39.

intoxication" when he "disturbed" the last meeting of the society with an "indecorous and untimely speech." [26] In expelling respected and competent homeopaths simply because of their different medical practices, the society placed them in a class with men like Kittredge, who deserved censure.

Although the dismissal of homeopaths from an orthodox society was an unhappy episode in the history of American medicine, it was an act which easily can be understood. The orthodox profession equated homeopathy with quackery. It seemed utterly ridiculous that anyone could believe in the efficacy of infinitesimals. Since the theory was so "absurd," anyone practicing it could be only a fraud or a fool. There was no place in serious medical convocations for frauds or fools. How, the allopaths asked, could any serious physician consult with a mere pretender? The homeopaths, moreover, treated according to a preconceived formula which did not always work. Yet they claimed that homeopathy was the *only* law of cure, and they rejected the orthodox treatments. Since the allopaths were firmly convinced that the homeopaths were deluded, it was only natural to deny them all access to professional society.

The battle between right and wrong is often difficult to resolve, but it is almost impossible to resolve the conflict between right and right. The allopaths were correct in refusing to consult with men whom they considered fools or knaves. On the other hand, the homeopaths could hardly be blamed for having adopted a system which they found superior to the orthodox practices. Neither could the regulars be criticized for expelling "deluded" men from their ranks. Could the homeopath be accused of having tested novel theories? Unless the orthodox medical profession was willing and able to provide a testing ground for innovation, it had to be done outside the allopathic institutions. There was truth on both sides in the conflict, yet at the same time both sides were "deluded."

The high point of intolerance came not with the expulsion of irregulars, but with the treatment of orthodox practitioners accused of having consulted with irregulars. For instance, on the night of the assassination of Abraham Lincoln, Secretary of State William Seward was stabbed three times in an attack upon his life. Dr. Tullio S. Verdi, a homeopath and Seward's family physician, joined Surgeon-General Joseph K. Barnes and several other doctors in a successful attempt to save the secretary. Later, Verdi wrote that the consultation was characterized by courtesy. "Not one

[26] Massachusetts Medical Society, Records of Boards of Trial, 1858–1881, pp. 174–93.

86

descended to that petty professional pique or ill-conceived pride of many practitioners, in reference to associating with a medical gentleman of a different school of therapeutics."

Intelligent men could find nothing objectionable in attending to the critically wounded, especially in the case of a leading government official. Yet, a vice president of the American Medical Association, Ohio's Dr. William H. Mussey, demanded that Barnes be severely censured for "allowing a quack to prescribe medically, whilst he was attending surgically." Mussey's accusation was discussed at the Boston meeting of the A.M.A. Dr. J. J. Woodward, of the United States Army, explained that Verdi had been Seward's family physician and that regardless of the ethical problem, if Barnes had not taken action, the secretary of state might have died. The delegates were satisfied with that explanation, and the matter was dropped.

Mussey, however, was not one to let such an obvious violation of medical ethics be forgotten. He called upon the Ohio State Medical Society to censure Barnes for his indiscretion. Like the A.M.A., the Ohio society refused to appear ridiculous by condemning the physician who had saved Seward's life. According to Mussey, the surgeon-general had acted unprofessionally when he rushed to aid the fallen secretary. Rather than lowering himself by consulting with a homeopath, Barnes should have allowed the ailing Seward to take his chances with homeopathic treatment.[27]

In a much more publicized case, six years later, the Medical Society of the District of Columbia refused to admit Dr. Christopher C. Cox. He was charged with having committed a grave offense against the code of ethics. He had served upon the same board of health as a homeopath, again Dr. Verdi. The *New York Times* commented in an editorial entitled "A Medical Absurdity." It noted that allopaths were terribly intolerant of homeopaths. "There is no stronger tenet in the orthodox creed than that it is better the patient should die under the old remedies than recover under homeopathic treatment." To further complicate matters, the Society had petitioned the House of Representatives, demanding that Verdi be replaced by a physician acceptable to the orthodox profession. The board of health replied with a series of resolutions to the effect that the divergent systems of practice had no relation to the work of the individuals serving on the board. "An educated homeopathic physician," it asserted, was "fully as

---

[27] *Western Homeopathic Observer* (St. Louis) 2 (May 15, 1865): 81–86; *Transactions of the A.M.A.* 16 (Philadelphia, 1866): 51–52; *Transactions of the Twentieth Annual Meeting of the Ohio State Medical Society* (Cincinnati, 1865), p. 7.

competent to judge of and direct the rules of hygiene as a graduate of any other school of medicine."[28]

Documents indicate that the violation of the consultation clause was merely a pretext for the action of the District of Columbia Medical Society. The Cox affair can only be understood in its relation to events of the previous years. In 1869 the Society had refused to admit Negro physicians. Furthermore, by a strange "sleight-of-hand," it had managed to establish a subsidiary, the Medical Association of the District of Columbia. The Association had rules and regulations which were contrary to the charter of the Society. The Association, for instance, could regulate the practice of medicine by prohibiting consultation with nonmembers. Since most fellows of the Society were also members of the Association, those not admitted to the Association found themselves denied all professional intercourse. Moreover, the Association only admitted those who were considered acceptable by the Society. The net result was that while Negroes were licensed by the Society, their inability to join the Association prohibited all consultation with white practitioners.

On January 3, 1870, the Society defeated a resolution providing that "no physician, who is otherwise eligible, shall be excluded from membership in this Society on account of race or color." The Society then reorganized the committee that had reported favorably upon the applications of three Negro physicians. The new committee was a "safe one," with one member "a doctor lately in the rebel service."[29] Drs. Christopher C. Cox and D. W. Bliss decided to take action to ensure the complete integration of Negroes into professional society. They founded the "National Medical Society of the District of Columbia," which immediately admitted the three Negroes. Cox and Bliss then tried to convince Congress to annul the charter of the original society.

Senator Charles Sumner, the radical Republican from Massachusetts, adopted the cause of the Negro physician as his own. Sumner's committee on the District of Columbia reported favorably upon Senate bill 511, which would have annulled the charter of the Society. The committee was satisfied that Negroes were excluded from the Society simply because of their color.

[28] *New York Times*, July 11, 1871, p. 4, cols. 4–5; *Hahnemannian Monthly* 6 (April 1871): 471; (June 1871): 555; (September 1871): 82–84. See also the *Medical and Surgical Reporter* (Philadelphia) 24 (June 3, 1871): 465–66.

[29] Samuel C. Busey, *Personal Reminiscences and Recollections of Forty-Six Years' Membership in the Medical Society of the District of Columbia . . .* (Washington, D.C., 1895), pp. 245ff.; *Senate Report Number 29*, 41st Cong., 2d sess., (Washington, D.C., 1870).

In the report, Sumner compared the Society to Rip Van Winkle: "The Medical Society act as if slavery still ruled, with its proscriptions, exclusions and tyrannies. Evidently they knew not that great sway of equal rights which has been declared." The committee urged that Congress withdraw its sanction from the Society.[30] Congress, however, refused to take action in the medical dispute.

Bliss and Cox took the affair to the American Medical Association. When the District of Columbia Medical Society selected its delegates to the 1870 convention, it made certain to exclude the "hostile faction," those who belonged both to the Society and the "National Society." The result was that the A.M.A. was faced with two sets of delegates from the District. After a great deal of discussion, the A.M.A. finally decided to exclude members of the "National Society." Thus, the Negroes and their supporters were not admitted to the 1870 convention. The A.M.A. action was not entirely unwarranted. The new society had acted quite unethically in trying to convince Congress to destroy the original one. In any case, the effect of the A.M.A. action was to reject Negro practitioners.[31]

The members of the D.C. Medical Society, however, were outraged at Cox and Bliss for daring to question the right of the Society to send delegates to the national convention. When Cox applied for membership in 1871, the Society was overjoyed at the opportunity to reject him. The stated reason for his rejection was his position on the board of health with Dr. Verdi, but in reality he was rejected because of his role in the 1870 integration attempt.

Bliss paved the way for his own expulsion when he openly challenged the Society. He announced that he had consulted with Cox at the bedside of Vice President Schuyler Colfax. That, of course, was contrary to the rules and regulations of the Medical Association of the District of Columbia, as Cox was not a member. In his reply to the formal charge, Bliss admitted that he had consulted with Cox and that he had also met professionally with Dr. Augusta, one of the Negro physicians who had been rejected by the Association. Now the Society had a reason to expel Bliss. They initiated charges against him for having violated the consultation clause by meeting with nonmembers of the Association. Bliss was summarily dismissed.

Bliss and Cox were rejected or expelled for having violated the consulta-

---

[30] *Senate Report Number 29*, pp. 5–6; see also John B. Nicholas, W. J. Mallory, and J. S. Wall, *History of the Medical Society of the District of Columbia, 1833–1944* (Washington, D.C., 1947), p. 30.

[31] *Transactions of the A.M.A.* 21 (Philadelphia, 1870): passim.

tion clause, but they were really being dismissed for their actions during the 1870 episode. At that time, Bliss had been a very popular physician; he had a large clientele of prominent public figures. James Garfield wrote to him that he noticed that the medical profession had "decorated" him with their censure. Garfield said: "I have no doubt it will do you good."[32] Bliss found to his great disappointment, however, that his case load dwindled until he could hardly support his family. At that point, in 1876, he apologized to the Society and asked to be readmitted. By a vote of 31 to 1, he was elected to fellowship. Cox followed the same course, in 1877, when he was admitted by a vote of 52–9.[33]

In the District of Columbia, the use of the consultation clause was merely a pretext for expelling "traitors" from the local Society. In Connecticut it was to have a more fatal effect. A New London homeopath was attending a difficult obstetrical case. When he decided that a specialist was required, he found that it was impossible to locate one willing to consult with irregulars. One allopath, declaring that "oil and water will not coalesce," refused to assist. Another old school doctor was summoned from Norwich. Before he could reach the bedside of the patient, however, an orthodox practitioner convinced him that he should not violate professional ethics. Honor was more valuable to the allopath than the life of a patient. When the homeopath could get no help, the patient finally died, a victim of the consultation clause.[34]

The height of absurdity was attained in 1878. The *New Haven Journal and Courier* printed a letter from "Patriot," which demonstrates the lengths to which the orthodox profession would go in their denunciation of homeopathy. A Norwalk physician, Dr. Moses B. Pardee, had been expelled from the Fairfield County Medical Society for having consulted with his wife, Dr. Emily V. D. Pardee, a homeopath. The writer noted sarcastically: "Had his offense been a bank defalcation, or had he consulted with another man's wife upon topics not purely medical, there is no reason to fear, as the times go, that his error might have been overlooked, or, at least, condoned." It was reassuring, he declared, "to find a body of men of stern integrity and inflexible purpose who will give to such a crime, perhaps I should say out-

---

[32] *Hahnemannian Monthly* 6 (September 1871): 82–84; Busey, *Personal Reminiscences*, pp. 274–87; Garfield to Bliss, Hiram, Ohio, July 13, 1871, in Garfield letter book, Library of Congress.

[33] Busey, *Personal Reminiscences*, pp. 290–93.

[34] *Norwich Bulletin*, cited in *New England Medical Gazette* 13 (July 1878): 318–19.

rage, as this, the swift condemnation and punishment it so richly deserves."[35]

There were also several cases in which respected allopaths were censured by their colleagues for having assisted irregulars in other ways than through professional consultation. One of those cases involved Dr. Henry A. Martin, a Boston surgeon. In 1868 he had been appointed a one-man committee on vaccination and was ordered to report from time to time on that subject to the delegates of the American Medical Association. Deciding that it was important to spread the knowledge of vaccination to all interested physicians, Martin submitted an article to the *New England Medical Gazette*, a homeopathic journal.[36] Martin's allopathic brothers were outraged at the vision of an allopath assisting the enemy. At the 1871 A.M.A. convention, he was severely rebuked for his indiscretion and relieved of his committee assignment, simply because he believed that the benefits of vaccination could not be restricted to the orthodox school. Supposedly, the science of medicine would be advanced if homeopaths were kept unfamiliar with vaccination.[37]

The attempts to enforce the consultation clause of the A.M.A. code of ethics did not destroy or even temporarily delay the progress of homeopathic medicine. If anything, persecution strengthened the will of the martyrs. It provided them with the moral assurance that they had something worth fighting to preserve. In addition, it brought them the sympathy of a public which cared little about medical theory. The orthodox profession had attempted to intimidate the sectarian by refusing to accept him as a worthy comrade, implying that he was totally incompetent. That attempt had failed in every particular. To be sure, some homeopaths were expelled from the allopathic fraternities. Those men, however, continued to adhere to their homeopathic views with even more tenacity. Moreover, the censure of leading allopaths like Drs. Augustus K. Gardner, Henry A. Martin, and Christopher C. Cox only made the press and public even more suspicious of the orthodox profession. The absurdity of the consultation clause issue, as exemplified in the Bliss–Cox affair and in the censuring of Cox for having served on the same board of health as an irregular made the orthodox profession appear in an even worse light. The consultation clause

---

[35] *New Haven Journal and Courier*, cited in *New England Medical Gazette* 13 (July 1878): 315–17; *Homeopathic Times* 7 (May 1879): 37–38.

[36] *Transactions of the A.M.A.* 19 (Philadelphia, 1868): 40; *New England Medical Gazette* 6 (January 1871): 27–32.

[37] *Transactions of the A.M.A.* 22 (Philadelphia, 1871): 24.

obviously could not effect the destruction of homeopathy. All that it accomplished was to bring public ridicule upon the profession.

It was clear that medical ethics left much to be desired. The code protected neither the conscientious physician nor his patient. Was a doctor being true to the oath of Hippocrates when he refused to assist an injured or diseased patient? While doctors were arguing the intricacies of medical ethics, the patient might die for lack of assistance. Moreover, the physician who was interested in the welfare of his patient was threatened with loss of professional recognition. Eventually a change had to be made. The consultation clause was ineffective in stemming the tide of homeopathy, and either the clause or the attitude toward irregular practitioners would have to be altered. A giant step toward resolving the crisis of ethics was to come as a result of events occurring at the University of Michigan.

VII

THE ANN ARBOR IMBROGLIO

AFTER THE ARRIVAL of the first homeopath in Michigan in 1843, the new system slowly gained in strength and numbers. As was the case in Ohio, New York, and elsewhere, the cholera epidemic of 1848 to 1852 created the opportunity for a comparison of homeopathic therapy with heroic medicine. As noted earlier, when the homeopathic treatment of that disease proved more effective than the allopathic remedies, homeopathy quickly gained public support. By 1851 the new school was so firmly entrenched that its advocates were able to convince the state legislature to repeal the medical license law and remove the implied inferiority.[1]

Even while the homeopaths were winning their first victory, they began to shift their attention to the problems of medical education. Rather than having to support their own college, they insisted that homeopathy be taught at the tax-supported University of Michigan. On April 8, 1851 the legislature enacted a statute providing for the addition of a homeopathic professor to the Ann Arbor faculty. The university regents, however, refused to let the legislators determine educational policy and took no action. In 1855 an almost identical bill again ordered the regents to appoint a homeopathic professor.[2]

Although the college was still allopathic, the delegates to the 1855 A.M.A. convention were horrified at the possibility of homeopathic "quackery" being taught at an orthodox school. On May 4 Dr. J. L. Atlee,

---

[1] Madge E. Pickard and R. Carlyle Buley, *The Midwest Pioneer: His Ills, Cures, and Doctors* (Crawfordsville, Indiana, 1945), pp. 216–17; see also Charles E. Rosenberg, *The Cholera Years* (Chicago, 1962), pp. 161–64.

[2] University of Michigan, *Proceedings of the Regents, 1837–1864* (Ann Arbor, 1915), pp. 604, 606, 608.

a Pennsylvania physician, rose to offer a resolution. "Any such unnatural union," he declared, "cannot fail" to "impair the usefulness of teaching" to such an extent that any school teaching two systems of practice would be unworthy of "the support of the profession." Dr. Alonzo B. Palmer, a professor at Ann Arbor, rose to second the motion. The censure was directed at the legislators who had "intruded" a chair of homeopathy, rather than at the unwilling faculty, and the proposal was adopted unanimously.[3]

The action of the A.M.A. was unnecessary since the Michigan regents had refused to appoint a homeopathic professor. From 1855 to 1866 the situation remained unresolved, despite strong pressure from the assembly. Finally, in 1867 the legislature passed a bill intended to force the regents to act. This measure requiring the introduction of homeopathy was attached to a university appropriation bill. The school would receive the proceeds of a property tax on the condition that the regents appoint a homeopath to comply with the law of 1855. At this point, more was involved than a medical dispute. When the legislators tried to dictate educational policy by withholding school funds, they were infringing upon the authority of the regents. Jealous of their prerogatives, the regents refused to let themselves be bribed into hiring anyone. Since the university was in severe financial straits, they sought a solution which would release the funds while ensuring their own independence.[4]

The faculty reaction to the dilemma was predictable. On February 20, 1867 Professor Palmer wrote to Edward C. Walker, an influential regent. As an allopath, Palmer was appalled at the thought of the university teaching both homeopathic and "scientific" medicine. He recognized that since the state had been subsidizing an orthodox school, it had the right to establish and support a homeopathic one. But such an institution, he said, should be located as far as possible from Ann Arbor.[5]

Another professor, Corydon L. Ford, informed Walker that the "true interest of the university" could only be advanced by the rejection of the appropriation and "its obnoxious conditions." He said that if the regents complied with the provisions of the 1867 law, the college would be disgraced in the eyes of the entire medical profession. "Presbyterian Prince-

[3] *Transactions of the A.M.A.* 8 (1855): 55.

[4] *Peninsular Journal of Medicine* 11 (December 1875): 551–62; Michigan Homeopathic Medical School Papers, petitions to regents, 1866–1867, Michigan Historical Collections, Ann Arbor.

[5] Palmer to Walker, Ann Arbor, February 20, 1867, Walker Papers, Michigan Historical Collections.

ton," he exclaimed, would not be more scandalized if an atheist was appointed to the chair of theology. Ford declared that he could not teach at any school which "gives official recognition to any System which the Medical Profession cannot recognize."[6]

When the regents convened on April 9, Professors Abram Sager and Silas H. Douglass joined Alonzo Palmer in denouncing the prospect of a homeopathic division within the medical department. Regent Walker had been considering the alternatives. If a homeopathic professor were appointed, it might lead to the resignation of the entire allopathic faculty. In that case, the addition of homeopathy would nullify the years of work involved in building the steadily improving institution. On the other hand, rejection of the legislative demand would jeopardize the finances of the entire university. At the April 10 meeting of the regents, Walker announced that homeopathic instruction at an orthodox college would not result in a "proper development of the principles and practice of Homeopathic Medicine." The wisest plan, he said, would be to construct a separate homeopathic school. In that way, the homeopaths would be satisfied with state recognition and support, while the allopathic college would not be threatened with destruction.[7]

Although Walker's plan was indeed a wise one, it was contrary to the ideas of an influential homeopathic faction. That group, led by Drs. A. I. Sawyer and S. B. Thayer, was convinced that the time had come for the orthodox profession to familiarize itself with homeopathy, as well as to teach it in allopathic schools. Sawyer and Thayer, therefore, denounced the regent's proposal, insisting that homeopathy be added to the Ann Arbor curriculum, as ordered by the legislature.

Another regent, T. D. Gilbert, was outraged at the intransigence of the homeopaths. He complained that in their quest for equality they were willing to "sacrifice every department of the university." They thought nothing of "placing themselves between the University and its much needed aid." Gilbert's wrath was not restricted to the homeopaths, however; he berated the faculty, too, asserting that the orthodox profession was guilty of "bigotry and intolerance." If the allopaths would only accept sectarianism, the regents would be able to appoint a homeopath and gain the appropriation.[8]

[6] Ford to Walker, Brunswick, Maine, March 8, 1867, ibid.
[7] University, *Regents Proceedings, 1864–1870* (Ann Arbor, 1870), pp. 197–98, 200.
[8] Gilbert to Walker, Grand Rapids, Michigan, July 18, 1867, Walker Papers.

In an editorial entitled "The Medical College Imbroglio," the *Michigan Argus* declared that the two rival systems could not exist side by side.[9] Dr. E. O. Haven, the university president, agreed with this sentiment. In a report to the regents, he noted that the state supreme court had decided that the plan to locate a homeopathic division away from Ann Arbor was not in compliance with the 1867 law. The appropriation, then, remained in the state treasury. Disregarding the school's financial difficulties, Haven argued that homeopaths should never be appointed. In the first place, he said, there never had been a professor of allopathic medicine. "What we want in the Department of Medicine and Surgery," he went on, "is a number of Professors who shall present all the *subjects* and all the *information* properly belonging to the science and art of Medicine and Surgery." Furthermore, the regents should be free to select the best qualified men, "untrammeled by the dictation of any bodies or parties of men outside of the University." We will not select teachers, Haven exclaimed, who would be "partisan defenders of exclusive theories;—as, for instance, in the Literary Department, Professors of Protestantism"; or in the Law department, professors of conservatism, radicalism, or democracy.[10]

By March of 1868 the regents realized that unless they acted soon the appropriation might be lost. Casting aside the opposition of Sawyer and Thayer, the board offered to establish the "Michigan School of Homeopathy" in some city other than Ann Arbor. The plan called for the appointment of only two professors, certainly not enough to operate a separate college. It would seem to indicate that the regents were making the proposal with the expectation that it would be rejected by the legislature. The regents could then get out of their dilemma by acceding to the assembly and blaming the destruction of the college upon the stubborn legislators and the recalcitrant faculty. Rather than await such an outcome, on April 11 five professors submitted their resignations.[11]

The *Detroit Advertiser and Tribune* reported that the entire allopathic faculty would transfer to the recently established Detroit Medical College. On June 2 when the trustees of the new institution announced their faculty it included three of the former university professors, Drs. Samuel G. Armor, Ford, and Palmer. From the beginning in 1850, medical professors at Ann Arbor had been unhappy about the lack of clinical facilities in that town. The threat of homeopathy made Detroit seem even more attractive

[9] *Michigan Argus* (Ann Arbor), April 24, 1868, p. 2, col. 3.
[10] University, *Regents Proceedings, 1864–1870*, p. 284.
[11] Ibid., pp. 267–68.

to the dissidents. In any case, the advantages of Detroit over Ann Arbor soon became merely academic, for in June of 1868 the regents persuaded Ford and Palmer to remain at their posts, apparently by assuring them that a homeopathic school would not be located at Ann Arbor.[12]

Despite the demands of the legislature and the pleas of the Hahnemannians, the new system was not introduced into the curriculum. After their mass resignation, the faculty had been guaranteed that the regents would not appoint a homeopathic professor "unless compelled by law." Regent Gilbert was willing to yield to the legislators in order to have the appropriation released, but his colleagues were more adamant.[13] The situation was precarious. The appropriation was in the state treasury, and the assembly demanded that the regents comply with the law before the funds were distributed.

In 1868 the convention of the Michigan State Medical Society was called to order amidst the uncertainties at Ann Arbor. The session was opened on June 3, the day after the Detroit Medical College announced that Ford and Palmer would serve on its faculty. Dr. E. P. Christian, of Wyandotte, offered a resolution which asserted that it was insane to proclaim that because a "wild theory, an insane hypothesis," had many "apologists and patrons," it was "entitled to the same consideration and official recognition as legitimate science." He insisted that "the medical chairs should be filled by honest, capable and enlightened gentlemen." As it would be self-defeating to turn the college over to those "of inferior acquirements and capacity," Christian urged the professors to remain at their posts. The resolution was referred to a committee which, on the following day, submitted an adverse report. The committee believed that if required to work with "quacks," the faculty "could not consistently remain." Dr. Palmer, who had already resigned, rose to take the floor. His voice breaking with emotion, pausing to wipe away the tears welling in his eyes, he exclaimed that he had devoted the "best part of his life" to the University of Michigan. Yet he insisted that "no honorable man could affiliate with homeopathy."[14]

The regents continued desperately to seek a way to resolve the crisis. Gilbert was constantly at Lansing, where he lobbied for the repeal of the act of 1855. Writing to Regent Walker in February of 1869, he said that if the act could not be annulled it would be necessary to appoint an "en-

---

[12] Leslie L. Hanawalt, *A Place of Light: History of Wayne State University* (Detroit, 1968), pp. 46–47.

[13] Gilbert to Walker, Grand Rapids, May 1, 1868, Walker Papers.

[14] Michigan State Medical Society, *Proceedings, 1867–68* (Detroit, 1869), pp. 34–35, 39–41.

tirely new faculty who are not afraid of contamination."[15] From 1869 to
1872 the state capital was often filled with homeopathic and allopathic
practitioners, regents, professors, and interested laymen. The allopaths continued to advocate a homeopathic college situated in some other town.
Strangely, many homeopaths joined their orthodox colleagues in this demand. Dr. E. R. Ellis, for instance, secretary of the Detroit Homeopathic
College, wanted his school to become the homeopathic branch of the state
university. Public support would have eliminated the financial difficulties
of his small sectarian college. Moreover, Detroit's homeopathic professors
sought the added prestige which accompanied positions with the state university.[16]

In a letter of December 1872 Thayer, a leader in the fight to add homeopathy to the Ann Arbor curriculum, described the factions involved. In
his manuscript on the history of homeopathy in Michigan, Sawyer also
assessed the situation. From these two sources, a clear picture emerges.
Dr. Ellis tried to convince the assembly that the homeopathic branch of
the university should be in Detroit, a city abounding in clinical material.
He argued that the state could save money by developing the Detroit
Homeopathic College, his own institution. At the same time, Drs. C. J.
Hempel, E. A. Lodge, and E. H. Drake proposed that the college be located
in Michigan's second largest city, Grand Rapids. In that case, they would
be able to join the faculty and add to their names the title "Professor."[17]

Relations between the various homeopathic factions became quite bitter.
Indeed, the acrimony between homeopaths seemed greater than that between homeopathy and orthodoxy. In a letter to Sawyer, Thayer demonstrated how vicious those relations had become. He commented upon
Lodge's "insolence and falsehoods" in his drive to unite homeopathy
behind the projected college at Grand Rapids. "If headed off in his
schemes . . . like a certain Squat animal we know of, he at once emits an
odor so suffocatingly offensive, that all who respect themselves, and the
profession to which they belong, are disposed to retire in disgust."
Lodge, he said, lies "with the glibness of a Falstaff, and rings Epithets like
a fisherwoman."[18]

[15] Gilbert to Walker, Grand Rapids, February 18, 1869, Walker Papers.
[16] Ellis to Walker, Detroit, May 21, 1873, ibid. See also J. D. Craig to A. I.
Sawyer, Niles, Michigan, July 28, 1869; and S. B. Thayer to Sawyer, Battle Creek,
January 9, 1870, in Sawyer Papers, Michigan Historical Collections.
[17] Thayer to Sawyer, Battle Creek, December 23, 1872, Sawyer Papers; see also
"Factions in Homeopathy in Michigan," ibid.
[18] Thayer to Sawyer, Battle Creek, June 21, 1869, ibid.

In 1873 the new president of the university, Dr. James B. Angell, agreed with his predecessor that legislative interference was to be avoided like the plague. Thayer and Sawyer had spent much of their time at Lansing, and in April the two homeopaths persuaded the assembly to enact yet another statute providing for the appointment of two homeopathic professors.[19] The regents again refused to act. The frustrated homeopaths and the irate representatives turned to the court. They applied for a writ of mandamus to force the regents to comply with the law. Once more, the court denied the motion.[20]

On April 24, 1873, the state senate "committee on sectarianism and homeopathy" convened at Ann Arbor to question the faculty. Ford admitted that he would not object to teaching anatomy to homeopathic students, unless, he said, his "professional friends should raise objections." Palmer declared that the introduction of homeopathy would prove disastrous to the college. Under the preceptor system, every student had to apprentice with a qualified practitioner. When the orthodox profession learned that homeopathy was taught at the school, he said, no respectable physician would send his students to the college. Moreover, the American Medical Association could be counted upon to exclude graduates who had associated with irregulars during their medical education. Palmer predicted that the addition of homeopathy would cause the school to sink into oblivion. Dean Abram Sager testified after Palmer, admitting that he knew absolutely nothing about homeopathy, but declaring that he was ready to take a firm stand against it.

Several homeopaths were present at the hearing. Dr. Ellis, of the Detroit Homeopathic College, provided some interesting information. He said that his school was founded in 1872, *with the encouragement of the regents.* Both he and the regents hoped that the Detroit College would eventually become part of the state university. This information helps to explain the actions of the board. The regents had always sought an alternate solution; Walker thought he had found it in a homeopathic division away from Ann Arbor. It appears that some action had actually been taken to that effect. In any case, Ellis continued his testimony by noting that the University was not as intolerant as it had been in the past. Two years before, the allopathic

[19] Angell to "My Dear Sir," Ann Arbor, March 31, 1873, in Angell Papers, Michigan Historical Collections; A. I. Sawyer, "History of Homeopathy in Michigan," pp. 543–44, MS in Sawyer Papers.
[20] 30 Mich. reports, 473; see also Burke A. Hinsdale, *History of the University of Michigan* (Ann Arbor, 1906), p. 144.

faculty had admitted one of his students, accepting a homeopathic certificate of two years of study.[21] Although much of the information given at the hearing helps to fill in gaps in the record, the testimony had no effect upon the situation. The legislature had already taken action, while the regents continued to seek a middle path.

On March 10, 1875, the medical faculty of the University of Michigan held a significant session. Drs. Douglass and Ford called the meeting, hoping to convince their colleagues to make concessions regarding the introduction of homeopathy. Douglass and Ford, who taught chemistry and anatomy, two noncontroversial fields, were willing to teach irregulars if that would prevent the dissolution of the school. They urged the faculty to stop resisting the legislative demands, because the state might withdraw financial support. It was better to admit homeopaths, they argued, than to let their own intransigence destroy the school. In the absence of any positive threat other than an unenforced law, the rest of the faculty refused to take action.[22]

The following month, April, the legislature again passed a bill providing for the appointment of a homeopath. This 1875 measure reflected the fact that the badly disorganized homeopathic profession had managed to achieve some semblance of unity. The Detroit Homeopathic College had merged with its Lansing counterpart, eliminating one faction. Then, on May 6, the Detroit school closed its doors so that its students could enroll at the state university.[23]

As in 1855, 1867, and 1873, the stage was set for the introduction of homeopathy into the university. The next move was up to the regents. At their May 11 meeting, Dr. C. Rynd rose to make a proposal. Rynd, a member of the board, was an allopath who was in favor of "some adjustment of the dispute between the rival schools of medicine."[24] Proposing that the act of 1875 be enforced, he recommended the establishment of a homeopathic college at Ann Arbor. According to his plan, two professors would be appointed to teach homeopathic therapeutics and *materia medica*. "Nonsectarian" fields, such as anatomy, physiology, and chemistry, would be taught by the allopathic faculty. The orthodox professors would examine and grade the class, including any homeopathic students. The diplomas

[21] *Michigan Senate Journal*, April 25, 1873, pp. 1991–2010.
[22] Minutes of the University of Michigan Medical Faculty, 1850–1875, MS in Michigan Historical Collections. See also *Detroit Review of Medicine and Pharmacy* 11 (March, 1876): 162–65.
[23] Sawyer, "History of Homeopathy in Michigan," pp. 644–62.
[24] B. F. Cooker to Walker, Ann Arbor, July 13, 1871, Walker Papers.

of the latter, however, would note their attendance at the homeopathic division.[25] The regents voted to adopt Rynd's proposal.

Now it was up to the faculty and the orthodox profession to react. On June 9 Dr. G. W. Topping offered a resolution to the Michigan State Medical Society. He repeated the familiar argument that the teaching of sectarian and orthodox medicine in the same school was "a scheme impossible to successfully carry out, and one fraught with disaster, and perhaps dishonor, to those who attempt its execution."[26] After a debate, the society decided to let the faculty handle the situation.

The faculty was in quite a bind. If the members resigned, they were handing the keys of the college to their most despised opponents. Moreover, they would appear foolish to a public which had always ridiculed the allopaths over the consultation question. The *Peninsular Journal of Medicine*, the organ of the faculty, believed that no "respectable set of doctors" could be found to replace a faculty which had resigned "upon such grounds."[27] In addition, it seems that the faculty was sick of the conflict and uncertainty of the previous eight years.

In any event, the *Journal* asserted editorially that the amalgamation plan was fully acceptable to the faculty. The two irregular professors would no more be an integral part of the medical school than were the departments of pharmacy or engineering. The editor suggested that far from being a disgrace, the introduction of homeopathy would sound the death knell of sectarianism. "So long as its champions were denied a place in the University, they appeared in the *role* of the persecuted." As a result, homeopathy had gained the sympathy of the public. Now that it would be taught at the school, it would "be obliged to stand on its own bottom—and," the editor chuckled, "a very infinitessimal [*sic*] bottom it is."[28]

Only one faculty member, the elderly and sickly Dean Sager, resigned his position.[29] When it was proposed, at a session of the Southern Michigan Medical Association, to censure the regents for having introduced homeopathy, Dr. Rynd, the regent whose accommodation with homeopathy resulted in the compromise, jumped to his own defense. If homeopaths were allowed to practice medicine, he said, they must be well educated. How,

---

[25] University, *Regents Proceedings, 1870–1876*, pp. 431–34. See also A. I. Sawyer, Diary, May 11–13, 1875, MS in Michigan Historical Collections.

[26] Michigan State Medical Society, *Transactions, 1875* (Lansing, 1875), p. 277.

[27] *Peninsular Journal of Medicine* 11 (November 1875): 538–39.

[28] Ibid. 11 (June 1875): 279–81.

[29] Michigan State Medical Society, *Transactions, 1876* (Lansing, 1876), p. 382; *Peninsular Journal of Medicine* 11 (June 1875): 275–77; (July 1875): 443–44.

he asked, could the profession justify the denial of a proper education to *any* physician? Under the plan, the orthodox faculty was not compelled to mix in any way with the homeopathic professors. Therefore, he said, condemnation of the regents was out of order. Rather, the regents should be complimented for their forward vision. The *Adrian Daily Times* reported that when Rynd had concluded his impassioned speech, he was "applauded vigorously" and the resolution was tabled.[30]

The reaction of the profession at large was different from that of the members of the Southern Michigan Medical Association. In August of 1875 the *Detroit Review of Medicine and Pharmacy* contained portents of things to come. Dr. William B. Atkinson, secretary of the American Medical Association, wrote to congratulate Sager for his correct and "manly stand." In the same issue, Dr. Leartus Connor, one of Detroit's leading physicians and an official of the Detroit Medical College, wrote that since the professors would be lecturing to irregular students, they would be serving on the homeopathic faculty. If the trend were not reversed, the eclectics, the hydropaths, and even the clairvoyants would be demanding their "rights." Connor condemned the "alliance of our medical schools with any form of quackery, even though the union be sugar-coated and infinitesimally diluted."[31]

A conflict was developing within the orthodox profession. Abram Sager, the resigned dean, immediately became the leader of those who denounced the faculty for remaining at their posts. In one of his frequent letters to the editor of the Detroit journal, Sager showed the inconsistency of the regular faculty. He noted their claim that "here and now are the time and place for the 'hand to hand' contest with the arch-enemy of rational medicine." Although the faculty seemed "already to anticipate a glorious triumph of arms, and even a Moody conversion of thousands of these obstinate heretics," he said, such a result was unlikely. According to the plan, the allopathic and homeopathic classes in *materia medica* and therapeutics were to be taught in different locations at the same time. How could the heretics be shown their errors, Sager correctly asked, when the irregulars would have no contact with the basic orthodox teachings?[32]

The "Independent Students" added their testimony to that of the former dean. They had been urged to help the faculty "combat Homeopathy in the University." So far, they said, "the 'combat' on the faculty side is a very quiet one." The "Students" proved their point by noting that Palmer,

[30] *Adrian Daily Times*, July 14, 1875, clipping in Angell Papers.
[31] *Detroit Review of Medicine and Pharmacy* 10 (August 1875): 505–10, 511–12.
[32] Ibid. 10 (November 1875): 674–76.

who had earlier spiced his lectures with denunciations of sectarianism, now was quite silent. The "doughty champion" of orthodoxy who had "led so many bloodless charges on homeopathic windmills, at a safe distance," had changed his tune. He "roars as mildly as a sucking dove, now that there is a brace of real live homeopathic professors in the medical department." Palmer had resigned in 1868 in order to prevent the introduction of homeopathy, but he later rejoined the faculty and remained at his post.

The "Independent Students" asserted, probably correctly, that in most cases the "combat" was decided in advance. Students in the homeopathic division had selected their system after several years with a preceptor who was a homeopathic practitioner. Regardless of the influence of the faculty, they would be homeopaths after graduation. The "Students" questioned the consistency of the faculty by noting that although irregular students were their classmates, after graduation they would no longer be considered fit for consultation. In conclusion, the "Students" declared that an excellent education was not enough, if they would forever be tainted by their affiliation with fledgling irregulars. "Our alma mater," they said, "must be like Caesar's wife, above suspicion." [33]

The unwillingness of the faculty to take action against homeopathy prompted the state society to take the initiative. In 1875 the society had decided to let the faculty handle the affair. The following year, the professors had not only taken no action, but they were teaching alongside two homeopaths.

At the 1876 convention, Eugene Smith, a Detroit practitioner, proposed that university graduates not be admitted to fellowship until some steps were taken against sectarianism. In response to Smith's motion, a nine-man committee was appointed to make recommendations, the first of which was an assertion that the situation was "not calculated to maintain or advance medicine as a science," nor was it "consistent with the honor or interests of the profession." The second resolution was a simple declaration that the state "cannot successfully teach either medicine or theology." Third, legislative "interference with the government of the University" was unconstitutional, "wrong in the principle and harmful in its results." Finally, the committee suggested that the society enroll neither sectarians nor graduates of any college "whose professors teach or assist in teaching" irregular medicine. [34]

Dr. George E. Frothingham, an Ann Arbor professor, rose in opposition. He asked how the faculty could have resigned without "disgracing them-

[33] Ibid. 11 (January 1876): 37–41.
[34] Michigan State Medical Society, *Transactions,* 1876, pp. 364–66, 381–84.

selves and casting a stigma upon medical ethics." Frothingham declared that if the society adopted the resolutions, it would lose the respect of all "civilized people." "Pass it," he exclaimed, "and if you can bear the infamy I can bear your censure." [35]

The first proposal, asserting that nonsectarian education was inconsistent with the honor and interests of the profession, was passed by a vote of 63 to 37. At that point in the proceedings, Dr. Donald McLean, a "tall, handsome blond Scotchman with a ruddy complexion," the professor of surgery, announced that the faculty was dissatisfied with the introduction of homeopathy, but that it was unable to determine a proper course of action. He said that he had sought the advice of Dr. Samuel Gross, the prominent and respected Philadelphia anatomist. Gross had urged McLean to remain at his post. The faculty had "the monster by the throat," Gross had said, "and if just left alone they will very soon have the satisfaction of strangling it." [36] After McLean had concluded his remarks, the second resolution, insisting that the state "cannot successfully teach either medicine or theology," was adopted by a large majority. The resolution, that "legislative interference with the government of the University" was "unconstitutional," was next to be passed. The final resolution, which censured the Ann Arbor faculty by refusing to accept their graduates in the state society, was tabled until the next session.

When the day's business had been completed, Frothingham and Rynd both announced their resignation from the society. Rynd complained that the convention was characterized by a "narrowness, bigotry, and injustice disgraceful to an honorable and learned profession." [37] Rynd's final comment referred to the belief that the Detroit Medical College had led the fight to destroy its competitor. Professor McLean, writing twenty years after the event, agreed that the officers of the "embryo weakling, the Detroit College of Medicine," had taken advantage of the Ann Arbor imbroglio in order to force the resignation of the faculty. In that way, the Detroit College could "be built upon its ruins." If McLean was correct, the Detroit College could be censured for seeking "to deliver the university into the hands of the irregulars." [38]

---

[35] Ibid., pp. 385–86.

[36] Ibid., pp. 386–92. The description of McLean is from Bertha Van Hoosen, *Petticoat Surgeon* (Chicago, 1947), p. 64.

[37] Michigan State Medical Society, *Transactions, 1876*, pp. 392–95.

[38] *Journal of the A.M.A.* 27 (August 22, 1896): 443–44; *New York Times*, May 14, 1876, p. 1, col. 6.

The Independence Day issue of the *Michigan Farmer* contained an editorial by Dr. C. H. Leonard, a Detroit physician who was later accused of animosity toward the Detroit Medical College. Leonard charged that the action of the society was intended to "kill" the medical school "in order that a rival medical college at Detroit might have a fuller sweep." The homeopathic question, he declared, was only a subterfuge.[39] Three weeks later, Frothingham informed the editor that two of the men who had drafted the four resolutions had confided to him that instead of fighting homeopathy, "they desired to destroy the Medical Department of the University." After several more weeks had passed, Frothingham named his two confidants, Drs. James A. Brown of Detroit, and Gerald K. Johnson of Grand Rapids.

Frothingham offered powerful evidence which indicates that he, McLean, Leonard, and Rynd were all correct in their assessment of the situation. In 1874 the state society had appointed a committee to prepare a medical licensure law. The committee had invited three homeopaths and three eclectics to participate in drafting the proposal. The bill which they produced would have created a nine-man board of censors, with representation in proportion to the strength of the sects. On March 25, 1875 the bill was finally enacted, providing for a board consisting of two members of each school of medical practice. That compromise was fully acceptable to the state society. These facts demonstrate that far from aiming to destroy homeopathy, the Michigan State Medical Society had been willing to consult with irregulars in order to regulate medical practice. Even more damaging was the fact that the society was willing to subject allopathic applicants to an examination by four irregular physicians. Since the society was not crusading against homeopathy, Frothingham insisted that it had intended to destroy the medical department of the university.[40]

Even if the society was using homeopathy as an excuse, the allopathic faculty still had to defend itself against the charges. Few delegates to the 1876 A.M.A. convention in Philadelphia knew anything of the motivation of the state society. They had heard enough when they were informed that orthodox professors were lecturing to sectarians. Dr. Joseph Toner, the medical biographer, proposed that physicians who "in any way aid or abet the graduation" of irregulars were doing so in violation of the spirit of the code of ethics. When the discussion degenerated into a question of exactly

---

[39] *Michigan Farmer*, July 4, 1876, p. 215, cols. 4–5.
[40] Ibid., July 25, 1876, p. 239, col. 5; August 15, 1876, p. 263, cols. 4–6.

what constituted "aiding and abetting" graduation, the A.M.A. judicial council was ordered to investigate the problem and submit a report at the next convention.[41]

In 1878 the Michigan State Medical Society met several weeks prior to the American Medical Association. Dr. E. Twiss charged that Alonzo Palmer, Donald McLean, Edward Dunster, and W. J. Herdman, all faculty members of the university, had violated the A.M.A. resolution by "aiding and abetting" the education of homeopaths. The society turned the problem over to its own judicial council, which reported that since Twiss had presented no evidence of an "overt act," the professors could not be punished.[42]

The spirited debate was resumed at the state convention. Dr. William Brodie, an exceptionally tolerant Detroit physician, asserted that if the professors taught homeopathy, they should be disciplined. But how, he asked, could any harm be done by "teaching regular medicine." Brodie compared the Ann Arbor dispute to a ridiculous religious situation. Could Reverend George Duffield, the Lansing minister, be accused of violating the tenets of his church because he preached "his doctrine of religion" to disbelievers who happened to be in the congregation? Brodie provoked an outburst of hissing from his colleagues when he declared in conclusion: "If there had never been any rivalry in teaching medicine in this state, the question would never have come up."[43]

After several physicians had condemned the faculty for educating irregulars, Donald McLean took the floor. He said that if the society so desired, he would resign his position. The professor of surgery insisted that orthodoxy could not help but profit from the situation. Those who were afraid of homeopathic gain, he said, were men of little faith. Truth could stand comparison. Replying to the charge that the homeopaths had been accepted as colleagues, McLean replied that the "janitor will not speak to the janitor of the Homeopathic college."[44] When the debate was concluded, the delegates voted on the fourth resolution, which was carried over from 1876 and virtually ignored in 1877. As noted earlier, this proposal denied membership to any graduates of any school "whose professors teach or assist in teaching irregular medicine." The resolution was finally rejected by a vote

[41] *Transactions of the A.M.A.* 27 (1876): 48.
[42] Michigan State Medical Society, *Transactions, 1878,* pp. 225–26.
[43] Ibid., pp. 200–3.
[44] Ibid., pp. 212–13.

of 62 to 42. Interestingly enough, the delegates with direct connections at the Detroit Medical College all voted against the Ann Arbor faculty.[45]

Less than three weeks after the state society had exonerated the professors, the dispute was taken to the American Medical Association. Dr. Edward Dunster, professor of obstetrics at the university, was selected as a delegate to the 1878 convention at Buffalo. The state society came under sharp attack for having nominated a man who was known to be "aiding and abetting the graduation" of sectarians. Dr. N. S. Davis, a founder of the A.M.A. and perhaps its most influential member, reported that although Dunster's actions were beneath the dignity of the profession, he was not in violation of any section of the code of ethics. After the delegates had been given an opportunity to condemn Davis for his inability to find some legal basis for the expulsion of Dunster, it was resolved that an amendment to the code was obviously necessary. An addition was drafted, but according to the by-laws it had to be held over until the next convention, so that the membership could study the proposed change.[46]

The autumn and winter of 1878 brought a great deal of excitement to the Ann Arbor campus. Early in November, there was a "murderous assault by a mob of medical students upon a houseful of women." In that case, the students gathered for what must have been an amusing if not educational raid upon a local brothel.[47] When the sensation had begun to subside, faculty disputes came to the fore. Dr. E. C. Franklin, the dean of the homeopathic division, accused Donald McLean of having neglected, abused, and threatened his homeopathic patients. A brawl resulted, with McLean, the younger of the two, striking the first blow. Franklin parried it and wrestled McLean to the floor. The two were separated when Franklin was beginning to choke his adversary.[48] Happily, that was apparently the first and last time that advocates of the two systems tried to settle their differences on a field of physical combat.

[45] Ibid., pp. 218–19. The four men were Drs. E. L. Shurley, J. H. Carstens, Eugene Smith, and Leartus Connor.

[46] *Transactions of the A.M.A.* 29 (1878): 39–40, 42; Morris Fishbein, *A History of the American Medical Association* (Philadelphia and London, 1947), p. 96. See also the interesting clipping from an unidentified newspaper, the *Times* (Chicago?), in scrapbook number one, Wayne State University Archives, Detroit.

[47] Minutes of the University of Michigan Medical Faculty, November 7, 1878; *Michigan Argus*, November 8, 1878, p. 3. See also the clipping from the *Detroit Evening News*, December 11, 1878, in scrapbook number one, Wayne State University Archives.

[48] *New York Daily Tribune*, December 10, 1878, p. 5, col. 5; *Michigan Argus*, December 20, 1878, p. 3; *Hahnemannian Monthly* 14 (February 1879): 107–8.

On May 7, 1879 the A.M.A. took up its amendment to the code of ethics. Edward Dunster prepared a speech in opposition to the change. At the same time, he defended himself against charges stemming from his service alongside homeopathic colleagues and his instruction of irregular students.

In his speech to the 1879 Atlanta convention, Dunster insisted that although he wanted to remain in the A.M.A., "not even membership would be a fitting price for the abandonment of scientific convictions." Medicine was always a "liberal profession," he said, and a "liberal profession" could not refuse to share knowledge and truth. Quoting from Thomas Cooley's *Treatise on Constitutional Limitations,* Dunster argued that the spirit of the law could never contradict the letter of the law. Therefore, if he had not violated the code of ethics, he could not have possibly violated its spirit. As long as the public insisted upon homeopathic practitioners, he said, it was the duty of the medical profession to see that they were as well educated as possible. Dunster went on to insist that upon that basis alone, it could not be illegal or unethical to participate in the education of future physicians.

The honor of a teacher depends not upon his audience, but upon his integrity and the truth of his teachings. How then, he asked, could the promulgation of scientific truth lead to the advancement of error? If applied to other professions, Dunster argued that the revision of the code would "prevent the professor of astronomy from teaching the Copernican system if among his students there were unbelievers who held to the Ptolemaic system." It would prevent the minister from preaching to any sinners, atheists, or heathen in his congregation.[49] If orthodoxy could not triumph in its competition with homeopathy, he exclaimed, "she deserves to fall and be buried in oblivion." Repeating the earlier words of Frothingham, Dunster asserted: "If you can stand the dishonor and discredit that must come with the adoption of this amendment, we certainly can stand your censure."[50] After he had completed his powerful and moving speech, the delegates decided that because of the small attendance at Atlanta, the proposal should be allowed to rest for one more year. Possibly, the strength of Dunster's convictions had persuaded so many members of their error that the opponents of homeopathy sought a reprieve.

[49] Edward Dunster, *An Argument made before the American Medical Association at Atlanta, May 7, 1879, against the proposed amendment to the code of ethics restricting the teaching of students of irregular or exclusive systems of medicine* (Ann Arbor, 1879), pp. 9–18.

[50] Ibid., pp. 21, 28.

At the 1881 meeting, in Richmond, the debate was resumed. By that time, Dunster's oration had been printed and widely distributed. It had convinced a great many physicians that the Ann Arbor faculty had been correct in their stand. A substitute amendment was adopted, which stated that no teacher should "examine or sign diplomas or certificates of proficiency" for irregular students.[51] After all the bitter fighting, the allopaths were allowed to continue to instruct homeopathic students, as long as they did not sign diplomas or certificates of proficiency. The faculty had been exonerated of all charges. At a meeting several weeks later, the dean of the college was instructed to relieve the orthodox professors of the obligation to sign all diplomas.[52] A subsequent entry in the minutes indicates that as late as 1886 the faculty was still granting certificates of proficiency to irregular students.[53] The A.M.A., however, was satisfied. Homeopathy continued to be taught at Michigan, and orthodox professors lectured to irregular students. The homeopathic problem had apparently been settled, both by the refusal of the faculty to turn the school over to their enemies, and by the inability of the A.M.A. or the state society to act against the professors.

[51] *Transactions of the A.M.A.* 32 (1881): 38–39.
[52] Minutes of the University of Michigan Medical Faculty, June 27, 1881.
[53] March 25, 1886, in ibid.

VIII

THE MEDICAL REVOLUTION

As NOTED IN CHAPTER ONE, during the 1860's and 1870's America's orthodox practitioners abandoned the harsh treatment of the age of heroic medicine. Blood-letting, blistering, leeching, cupping, sweating, and purging were gradually eliminated from the physician's armamentarium. In 1856 Dr. George B. Wood, president of the American Medical Association, told the delegates to the national convention that the homeopathic successes had played a major role in forcing the allopaths to reevaluate their techniques, thereby eliminating the more ineffective or harmful therapeutics. Hahnemann's main contribution, he said, was to demonstrate that "diseases often get well of themselves, if left alone."[1] As more and more doctors recognized that patients did recover faster and with less discomfort under mild remedies than under harsh orthodox treatments, heroic practice moderated.

In his article on the decline of venesection, Charles S. Bryan quoted several physicians who noted that by 1870 the lancet was considered by most doctors to be detrimental to the health of the weaker patients. Dr. Austin Flint, the prominent New York allopath, wrote in 1866 that the "infrequent use of the lancet now, contrasted with its frequent use twenty-five years ago, constitutes one of the most striking changes in the practice of medicine."[2] A Kansas doctor agreed with Flint when he asserted: "The

[1] *Transactions of the A.M.A.* 9 (1856): 64–66.
[2] Austin Flint, *A Treatise on the Principles and Practice of Medicine* (Philadelphia, 1866), p. 129, cited in Bryan, "Blood-letting," *Bulletin of the History of Medicine* 38 (1964): 521.

lancet has finished its course and been laid away in the grave as quietly as many of its former victims."[3]

In addition to the moderation of practice by experienced practitioners, medical schools ensured that younger doctors did not resort to the most heroic of remedies. Blood-letting was advocated only in cases involving inflammation or cardiac congestion, and in many schools the students were not given instruction in the use of the lancet. An examination of textbooks has indicated that after 1860 relatively few graduates were familiar with that age-old remedy.[4]

Eventually, even the use of the lancet in the treatment of inflammation came under attack. In 1866 Detroit's Dr. Theodore A. McGraw addressed the Wayne County Medical Society on the hazards of venesection in childhood diseases. Upon investigating, he had discovered that the three leading texts by Condie, Meigs, and West all prescribed "very heroic" treatment for inflammatory diseases. McGraw was appalled to learn that such reputable authorities still continued to advocate "violent" therapeutics. "Mere hydrolic [sic] pressure" could hardly cause inflammation, he said, so how could it be expected to relieve those symptoms? Moreover, blood-letting had never been clinically proven beneficial. McGraw called upon his colleagues to use the most modern statistical methods to scientifically evaluate the effects of heroic medicine on childhood ailments. Until the results of such a study could be published, the Detroit physician urged caution with a remedy which "might do as much harm as bleeding."[5] In 1867 the members of the Chicago Medical Society debated the question: "What is the practical value of blood-letting in the treatment of disease?" During the course of the discussion, three physicians argued against venesection in any illnesses; nine others recommended the lancet only in a few specific difficulties.[6]

Two years later, in an address to the Michigan State Medical Society, William H. DeCamp, a Grand Rapids physician, described the changes which had recently taken place in orthodox practice. Many of those in

[3] Thomas N. Bonner, *The Kansas Doctor* (Lawrence, 1959), pp. 20–21, cited in Bryan, "Blood-letting."
[4] Bryan, "Blood-letting," pp. 525–27. Also see Lester King, "The Blood-letting Controversy: A Study in the Scientific Method," *Bulletin of the History of Medicine* 35 (1961): 1–13.
[5] Theo. A. McGraw, "Treatment of Inflammatory Diseases of Children by Bleeding," *Detroit Review of Medicine and Pharmacy* 1 (November 1866): 337–42.
[6] Chicago Medical Society, minutes, May 17, 1867, MS in Chicago Historical Society.

attendance, the doctor said, could recall the time when remedies were so harmful that they could "destroy the comfort, if not endanger the life of the patient." DeCamp described "how enthusiastically" Professor Martyn Paine tried to convince his students at New York University of "the great power and efficacy of blood-letting in the treatment of every inflammatory disease, from infancy to extreme age." Yet, DeCamp asserted, such a change had occurred that now few doctors were foolish enough to let blood in any cases.[7]

By 1870, then, venesection was no longer employed by the vast majority of physicians, although a few prominent men still sought to convince their colleagues of the benefits of the lancet. Dr. Henry Ingersoll Bowditch, son of Nathaniel Bowditch, the respected astronomer and navigator, was among them. A specialist in chest diseases, he published a paper entitled "Venesection, its abuse formerly—its neglect at the present day." Although admitting that human life had been "shortened and certainly made more miserable" by massive blood-letting, Bowditch declared that a great many practitioners had produced instant relief of "violent, acute, cardiac disease" by a speedy resort to the lancet. In addition, discomfort from lung congestion always could be alleviated by venesection.

Proclaiming that "evil is good run mad," the Boston doctor insisted that blood-letting was an effective remedy which was overused in the past. Forty years ago, he said, it "was an unmitigated evil." It was so widely abused, so disgusting, and so often debilitating that reputable physicians discarded the lancet. The result, he declared, was that instead of indiscriminate bleeding, the American physician was "using other remedies with a recklessness quite equal to the venesection of former days." Patients were being injected with opiates and other narcotics. In addition, alcohol had become a remedy popular among doctors and patients alike. Bowditch predicted that the new practices would prove as detrimental as the "over-bleeding" of the past.[8]

The Boston doctor added to his comments the testimony of Benjamin Ward Richardson, one of Britain's leading sanitationists and a well-known physician and lecturer. Like Bowditch, Richardson was certain that blood-letting was so beneficial in specific ailments that it should not be allowed to disappear from the physician's repertoire. If venesection had never been practiced, he asserted, "were some man to discover it, we should receive

---

[7] Michigan State Medical Society, *Transactions, 1869* (Lansing, 1869): 1–7.
[8] Henry I. Bowditch, *Venesection, Its Abuse Formerly—Its Neglect at the Present Day* (Boston, 1872), pp. 6–7.

that man as the greatest amongst us and send him to posterity as one of the lights of the age."[9] Bowditch concluded his essay with the comment that fear of the lancet had "paralyzed" medical practice, preventing the recovery of patients who might be saved by the *"Rational Use of Venesection."*[10]

As noted by Bowditch, narcotics and alcohol replaced blood-letting and calomel during the 1860's. One homeopath, Dr. Joseph Hooper, insisted that the change was but a minor one. "The Old School practice was much more cruel and barbarous thirty years ago than it is now," he admitted. "Lancets, leeches, blisters, and fearful drastic purges were the order of the day. Every one expected when he sent for the doctor, to be tortured before he was cured." Although the modern doctor no longer bled and leeched his patients, Hooper insisted that "horrible, nauseous, debilitating doses of medicine are still given." "Oh Calomel! Morphine! Quinine! Are ye not as dreadful and almost as fatal as the plague?"[11]

Despite Hooper's condemnation of orthodox remedies, quite a revolutionary development had occurred. The lancet rested, and calomel, its deadly companion, was no longer considered a panacea. Milder medication replaced the drastic remedies of the early days. As time passed, more and more physicians placed less emphasis on therapeutics and relied upon the body's natural healing powers.[12] Although one set of dangerous remedies was at first replaced by an array of only slightly less harmful ones, the use of milder therapeutics was an impressive step toward modern medicine.

The allopaths were not the only American physicians to alter their practices. Almost as soon as homeopathy was introduced into America, its practices began to deviate from the tenets of Hahnemannian medicine. Many who considered themselves disciples of the German theorist repudiated aspects of the original system. Some renounced the doctrine of infinitesimals; they dispensed homeopathic drugs in large doses. Others began to employ orthodox treatments, administering "brisk" purges, prescribing calomel and alcohol, and at times even using the lancet.

Hahnemann's principles were abandoned for a number of reasons. In the first place, as graduates of orthodox medical schools, many homeopaths had experienced the benefits of various allopathic treatments. When the situation arose, it was natural for them to administer a time-tested remedy.

[9] *Practitioner*, (November, 1868), cited in ibid., pp. 29–30.
[10] Bowditch, *Venesection*, p. 33.
[11] *American Homeopathic Observer* (Detroit) 3 (1866): 85–86.
[12] For a comment on the passing of alcohol, see *New York Times*, November 13, 1898, p. 18, col. 4.

Then, too, many homeopaths were "eclectic." [13] Those who were originally allopaths had investigated homeopathy because of its promise of success. They could be expected to employ orthodox remedies which seemed especially useful, and they were well able to experiment with newer forms of treatment. A third factor was a desire for respect. Those homeopaths who hoped to remain within the organized profession could hardly espouse the doctrine of infinitesimals when it appeared totally ridiculous to the orthodox physicians.

A final explanation for the renunciation of homeopathy was that it was exceptionally difficult to become a competent Hahnemannian. The homeopath, for instance, had to take a more complete medical history of his patient. According to theory, he might have to treat an illness which had been suppressed years earlier. He also had to know the results of hundreds of drug provings, so he could prescribe a medicine which would cause the same "totality of symptoms" when given in large doses to healthy subjects. Finally, the disciple of Hahnemann had to recognize the need for higher potencies (dilutions) in order to use the correct dose. It was easier to be an orthodox practitioner. The allopath could rely upon a specific remedy for each ailment. It was so much more trouble, then, to practice according to Hahnemann, that many homeopaths began to simplify their work by employing orthodox remedies and by increasing dosage.

Two homeopaths, Drs. William H. Holcombe and J. C. Peterson, provide excellent examples of the sectarian dilemma. In 1852 Holcombe, a Louisiana practitioner, published a work entitled *The Scientific Basis of Homeopathy*. He said in it that he "was so dissatisfied with the loose statements, the hasty inferences, and the dogmatism" of Hahnemann's *Organon*, that he "dropped it at about the 200th page, and never finished its perusal." [14] A practicing homeopath, then, and one who was serious enough to write about his system, had renounced the ideas of the founder of his sect.

Peterson, a Canadian physician, wanted to be accepted by his allopathic colleagues, but without abandoning homeopathy. In order to gain professional respectability, he declared that homeopathy must purge itself "of all that borders upon the transcendental and mysterious." That meant, of course, eliminating the concept of infinitesimals and repudiating the idea

---

[13] Not to be confused with the medical sect known as "eclectics," who were basically progressive Thomsonians, men who encouraged education and a combination of allopathic remedies with botanicals.

[14] William Holcombe, *Scientific Basis of Homeopathy* (Cincinnati, 1852), p. 269.

that shaking the vial of medication spiritually altered its potency. The average orthodox practitioner had little respect for the physician who prescribed practically no medicine, especially at a time when allopaths were still administering relatively huge doses. Peterson urged his colleagues to adopt the more reliable orthodox practices. "If it is our duty to heal the sick," he said, "we should reject *no* means that would assist us in our undertaking. We are to give relief, and not to follow the iron dogma of any man, or sect of men." He suggested that the modern homeopath must be able to combine the best of the several systems into a safe and effective practice.[15]

In the following year, 1861, an Alabama homeopath agreed with Peterson when he rhetorically asked: "Is Hahnemann the Alpha and Omega of Homeopathy?" The founder of the system, he said, was only half right in his discoveries. The size of the dose was totally immaterial. Homeopathy, the southerner declared, must be re-defined to include only the law of similars.[16]

During the 1860's the homeopathic profession began to fragment over the desire of some practitioners to modify Hahnemann's practices and to rejoin their allopathic comrades. In 1861 Dr. John C. Peters publicized the rift when he announced his resignation from the editorial board of the *North American Journal of Homeopathy.* Declaring that he was "opposed to all exclusivism and one-sided-ism" in religion, politics, science, and his "much-loved profession," Peters renounced Hahnemannian medicine. He always had sought to incorporate allopathic advances into his homeopathic practice, he said, usually against the wishes of his friends who considered the German physician a medical savior.[17]

Peters explained his position in a letter to the *American Medical Times,* an orthodox journal edited by two New York physicians, Stephen Smith and George Shrady. He began by insisting that he did not "believe or practice according to any one medical dogma or exclusive system." Moreover, he admitted that he had never prescribed infinitesimal doses. The high dilution, he said, was "so repugnant to every fraction of common sense which I possess, that I have always felt absolutely degraded" when trying it. In fact, he was so convinced that he "was dealing with quantities so

---

[15] J. C. Peterson, "On the Dissension between the Schools," *North American Journal of Homeopathy* 9 (November 1860): 308–12.

[16] John H. Henry, "Is Hahnemann the Alpha and Omega of Homeopathy?" *North American Journal of Homeopathy* 10 (November 1861): 245–49.

[17] *North American Journal of Homeopathy* 9 (February 1861): 535–37.

minute and so powerless" that, as he exclaimed, "it would be trifling with the lives of my friends" to depend upon them in serious cases. He even repudiated the *similia*, which he declared to be a "mere fragment of the greater law." Since scientists must "prefer the greater to the lesser truth," Peters said that he was ready to rejoin the ranks of orthodox medicine.[18]

One allopath, who signed his letter to the *Times* "Contraria Contrariis," insisted that Peters should not be readmitted to professional society. Before he could be considered orthodox, "Contraria" demanded that Peters completely discard homeopathic remedies and consult with no irregular practitioners. The New York homeopath replied to the attack by declaring that "unlike Contraria," he could in good conscience sign the A.M.A. code of ethics, as he did not confine his practice to an "all-exclusive dogma."[19]

Within a year, three other New York homeopaths had followed Peters' example. Drs. Edward P. Fowler, William F. Browne, and W. O. McDonald informed the *Medical Times* that they were absolving themselves "from any and all medical sects." They insisted that since they were not dogmatic followers of Hahnemann, they should not be ostracized for an alleged association with an exclusive theory.[20]

Sharp divisions were appearing within organized homeopathy. The high-dilution advocates, who considered Hahnemann the "Messiah of Medicine" and who accepted his every word as a revelation from above, became known as "pure" homeopaths, or "Hahnemannians." In opposition to them were the "eclectic" homeopaths, those who accepted orthodox remedies or who dispensed homeopathic drugs in large doses. In 1871 one author, who examined homeopathy "as it was and how it is," estimated that of the 75 homeopaths in Chicago, only 8 or 10 could be considered "pure." Only 5 or 6 of those high-potency men were devoted followers of Hahnemann in every aspect of practice. The remainder were "eclectics" who dispensed allopathic drugs in allopathic doses.[21]

In 1873 five New York "eclectic" homeopaths announced that they were publishing a journal, the *Medical Union.* They hoped it would help to reunite the profession. Drs. Charles E. Blumenthal, Egbert Guernsey, John C. Minor, and Albert E. Sumner joined in the venture with Augustus K. Gardner, who earlier had been expelled from the New York Academy of

[18] *American Medical Times* 3 (August 17, 1861): 108–9.
[19] Ibid., 3 (September 7, 1861): 156–58; (October 5, 1861): 228–30; (October 26, 1861): 282.
[20] *Boston Medical and Surgical Journal* 65 (September 5, 1861): 108.
[21] Charles W. Earle, "Homeopathy as It Was and How It Is," *Chicago Medical Examiner* 12 (September 1871): 531–33.

Medicine. *Similia*, they said, was not the only law of medicine; it was only a "fact holding good in many instances." The five men wanted to be known as "physicians," rather than as homeopaths.[22]

The *New York Times* editorialized upon the attempt to reunite the nation's physicians. "Few have ventured to dream" that medical sectarianism would ever end, that the orthodox lion would "lie down, so to speak, with the homeopathic lamb." The struggle between the sects had been so vicious that scars remained on either side. While the allopath had "so often and so plainly proved the homeopathist to be the worst of quacks," the editor noted, the homeopath had equally shown his rival to be a "bigoted adherent of a system of exploded follies." Despite the difficulties of the past, the *Times* suggested that consolidation had been made possible by the evolution of allopathic and homeopathic practice. The homeopath "differs widely from the original disciples of HAHNEMANN." The modern homeopath, the editor asserted, was better educated and less dogmatic than the early convert from orthodoxy. At the same time, allopaths had abandoned heroic medicine. They had discarded the lancet and "grown less lavish in dispensing calomel." Professional unity was not only possible, the *Times* declared, but it was an action which "commends itself to common sense."[23]

In 1875 the New Jersey State Homeopathic Society discussed the problem of sectarianism in an age of scientific medicine. One physician, a Doctor Dennis, insisted that the profession should consist of "physicians," men who were "searching after truth, for the good of mankind." Dennis reportedly told his colleagues that "if he found plasters and blisters useful, he should use them." The more dogmatic Hahnemannians in attendance were quick to denounce the "apostacy" in his remarks. Others openly repudiated Hahnemann's teachings. Professor Lillienthal, for instance, upon being summoned to the bedside of a dying man, "suddenly made up his mind to bleed him." He proceeded to let blood until the patient was relaxed. "It might not have been homeopathic," he declared, but it was the correct remedy for that case.[24]

Two years later, the *New York Daily Tribune* asked why medical sectarianism was allowed to continue. It was unscientific, as well as detrimental to the public health and well-being. The editor illustrated the results of the

---

[22] See various numbers of the *Medical Union*, vols. 1 and 2 (1873–74) and the *North American Journal of Homeopathy*, n.s., 3 (February 1873): 421.

[23] *New York Times*, February 7, 1873, p. 4, col. 4.

[24] *New York Daily Tribune*, May 17, 1875, p. 6, cols. 3–4.

"unnecessary" professional dispute. An inmate of the Philadelphia Home
for Aged and Infirm Colored Persons "became a lunatic." Two homeopaths
certified to his insanity and wanted to remove him to the proper department
of the almshouse. Dr. Muller, an allopath, had to sign an authorization
for the transfer, and medical ethics reared its ugly head. He was afraid that
if he acted upon the advice of irregulars, he might be expelled from the
county medical society. While he hesitated, the patient "settled it, . . . by
jumping from a fourth-story window." The lesson that the allopaths should
learn from the case, the editor said, was that the homeopaths "at least
knew a lunatic when they saw him."[25]

A series of letters to the editors of the *New York Times* indicate that
homeopaths were trying to determine how to maintain their identity in a
world without heroic medicine. After all, they realized that it was the abuse
of venesection and calomel which enabled them to develop into a large and
respected school of medicine. Now that allopathic treatment had moderated,
many homeopaths recognized that their system was too dogmatic and un-
changing to survive in an age of science and discovery. The letter which
opened the discussion was written by "Medicus," a homeopath who had
renounced the infinitesimal. He noted that Dr. George Wyld, vice president
of the British Homeopathic Society, had informed Benjamin Ward
Richardson that the English homeopaths wanted to cast aside their sectarian
label. "Medicus" agreed with Wyld, declaring that Hahnemann's claims
were extravagant and often wrong. For three months, the *Times* editorial
office was flooded with letters commenting upon the changing medical
practices. The correspondence demonstrates that the homeopaths were
sharply divided between the purists and the "eclectics," but also that many
irregulars wanted to merge with the allopaths.[26]

Possibly in response to Wyld's letter to Richardson, in October of 1877
Philadelphia's Dr. Adolph Lippe, America's foremost Hahnemannian,
circulated a carefully prepared "Statement of the essential points of the
Homeopathic Doctrine." Lippe wanted his colleagues to read the tenets
of traditional homeopathy, and sign a "Declaration of Homeopathic
Principles." It actually amounted to a confession of faith, asking every

[25] Ibid., September 7, 1877, p. 4, col. 4.
[26] *New York Times*, October 10, 1877, p. 5, col. 2. See also October 14, p. 6,
col 7; October 21, p. 5, cols. 4–5; October 24, p. 2, col. 4; November 4, p. 5,
cols. 2–3; November 11, p. 2, cols. 2–3; November 18, p. 5, cols. 3–4; November
25, p. 5, cols. 4–7; December 2, p. 10, cols. 4–6; and December 9, p. 10, cols.
4–7.

homeopath to avow that the law of similars and the doctrine of infinitesimals were infallible guides. Dr. R. C. Sabin, a Milwaukee homeopath,
was outraged at the dogmatism and intolerance implied in Lippe's action.
He wrote to the editor of the *Homeopathic Times* to express his anger at
the "Homeopathic Gospel-according-to-Lippe." [27]

The Philadelphian defended his action by asserting that a "statement of
faith" was necessary when a leading British homeopath was proposing
union with allopaths, and when Dr. Horace M. Paine, an "eclectic," was
attacking the major concepts of his sect. Lippe insisted that a declaration
of faith would prevent the "perversion" of Hahnemannianism by the "pretending members of the homeopathic school." [28]

Lippe and several other high-potency advocates decided to establish a
journal which could advance their viewpoint. He, Dr. Samuel Swan of New
York, and two British homeopaths were soon publishing the *Organon*, an
Anglo-American venture. The stated intention was to repel the "advancing
stream of Anti-Hahnemannian 'Muscovites'" who sought to repudiate the
homeopathic heritage and rejoin the orthodox profession. The *New
England Medical Gazette* agreed with Lippe that the time had come for the
homeopaths to purge their ranks, but not in the way suggested by the
Philadelphian. The editor refused to let himself be judged by the ridiculous
cures claimed by the purists, and he practically advocated the liquidation
of the Hahnemannians. [29]

The *Homeopathic Times* agreed with the *Gazette*. It declared that the
dogmatism of the high-potency men "can hardly find a parallel in the
world's history," and would turn "the dial plate of time backward to the
darkness of the darkest ages." The "eclectics," the editor declared, would
prefer "being freemen, bound by the trammels of no sect." "If this is
treason," the *Times* exclaimed, "make the most of it." [30]

In 1878, the same year which saw the emergence of Lippe's *Organon*,
New York's homeopathic profession was wracked by internecine strife. As
early as December of the previous year, the Albany County Homeopathic
Medical Society passed a resolution which declared that the "theory of
dynamization of drugs promulgated by Hahnemann in the Organon is . . .
false in theory, and should be discarded by the homeopathic profession." [31]

[27] *Homeopathic Times* (New York) 5 (October 1877): 161–62.
[28] Ibid. (November 1877): 186–87.
[29] *New England Medical Gazette* 13 (March 1878): 118–23.
[30] *Homeopathic Times* 6 (August 1878): 115.
[31] Ibid. 5 (January 1878): 238.

A homeopathic society had thus rejected the necessity of following a main Hahnemannian tenet.[32] The Homeopathic Medical Society of Northern New York took a similar step. The members adopted a resolution which declared that "the use of remedies in Inappreciable Doses is Non-Homeopathic." In so doing, they renounced the infinitesimal dose.[33]

Other rumblings of discontent were coming to the surface. On February 8, 1878, the Homeopathic Medical Society of the County of New York passed a proposal declaring faith in the law of similars. It continued, however, to state that "this belief does not debar us from recognizing and making use of the results of any experience."[34] By this action, the society had voted to allow the use of allopathic as well as homeopathic remedies. Editorializing, the *Daily Tribune* suggested that since the homeopathic society had indicated that the two sects practiced similar types of medicine, they should unite. "The needs of the suffering patient should be more important to the doctor than the dogmas or the ethics of his school. His business is to save life, whether by the orthodox or the heterodox method."[35]

Dr. E. P. Fowler, one of the three homeopaths who in 1862 had disavowed themselves from their connection with organized sectarianism, went quite a bit further than most of his irregular colleagues. On April 10, 1878, he emerged as the leader of the drive to renounce the law of similars. Fowler proposed a number of amendments to the constitution of the New York county medical society. If they were adopted, members would no longer be required to restrict their practice to homeopathic treatment. Furthermore, fellowship would be open to any physician who "has given satisfactory proof . . . that he fairly understands the principles of homeopathy." To the Hahnemannians, this was the ultimate heresy. What did homeopathy mean, they asked, if the society did not require the practice of Hahnemann's system? In order to allow more intensive examination of the amendments, and possibly to prevent a secession vote on one side or the other, the proposals were tabled.[36]

That same year, 1878, while the New York society was trying to resolve the struggle between the high- and low-potency factions, the Illinois Home-

[32] Ibid. 5 (February 1878): 257–59.
[33] Ibid. 6 (November 1878): 197–98.
[34] *New England Medical Gazette* 13 (March 1878): 128.
[35] *New York Daily Tribune*, March 9, 1878, p. 10, col. 2; March 13, 1878, p. 4, col. 5.
[36] *New York Times*, April 11, 1878, p. 8, col. 2.

opathic Medical Association encountered the same problem. The Illinois homeopaths began by debating a motion which declared that *similia simili-bus curantur* was "the best general guide in the selection of remedies." The members were asked to swear that they "fully intend to carry out this principle to the best of [their] ability." The "eclectic" homeopaths managed to append to the resolution a statement that since the welfare of the patient must always be uppermost in the mind of every physician, any necessary treatment could be employed. The revised proposal offended the Hahnemannians, who refused to admit that orthodox medicine was beneficial in the slightest degree. Since the amended resolution satisfied neither the high- nor the low-potency factions, it, too, was tabled.[37]

In 1880 the homeopathic profession formally separated into the two major groups. At the Milwaukee meeting of the American Institute of Homeopathy, the purists denounced the ideas of their more liberal colleagues. Declaring that Hahnemann's *Organon* was "the only reliable guide in therapeutics," they established the International Hahnemannian Association (I.H.A.). "WHEREAS, Numbers of professed Homeopaths not only violate these tenets, but largely repudiate them; and WHEREAS, An effort has been made on the part of such physicians to unite the Homeopathic with the Allopathic school," it was time, they exclaimed, that "legitimate Hahnemannian Homeopaths should publicly disavow all such innovations." By 1881, fifty-nine high-potency men had shown their disdain for the "eclectics" by signing the original membership list of the International.[38]

The formation of that Association led to an even greater polarization of the homeopathic profession. The minority, the purists, had grown more dogmatic in reaction to the liberalism of the majority. The quarrel within the ranks of the homeopaths became even more bitter. The *North American Journal of Homeopathy* asked of the Hahnemannians: "are these men knaves or fools? Can their cures be believed and their examples followed, or are they the emanations of diseased brains?" The "eclectic" faction was embarrassed when the high-potency advocates reported fantastic cures, effected by remedies so highly diluted as to make the claim appear fanciful. "When we present these reputed cures as homeopathic," the *Journal* said, "we do that which has no foundation other than the fertile imagination of

---

[37] Gonzalvo C. Smythe, *Medical Heresies: Historically Considered* (Philadelphia, 1880), pp. 160–66.

[38] International Hahnemannian Association, list of members, 1881, MS in Hahnemann Medical College Library, Philadelphia, Pennsylvania.

the author." It concluded: "We deny to the I.H.A. the satisfaction to excommunicate us, for we consider ourselves honest and upright followers of Hahnemann."[39]

Many allopaths recognized that homeopathy had undergone substantial changes over the years. In 1881 C. A. Devenport, a professor at the Michigan College of Medicine, urged his orthodox friends to consult with homeopaths. They differ, he said, "very little from the advanced disciples of our own school." Moreover, consultation could result in the destruction of sectarianism, as physicians of each school would learn of the benefits of the other. "Let us not be too arrogant," he declared. No school of medical practice "can possess all the truth; no system or school be entirely without error."[40]

Several years later Dr. H. C. Wood, a long time editor of the *Philadelphia Medical Times* and a professor at the University of Pennsylvania Medical School, told a convocation at Yale University that neither allopathy nor homeopathy was the "whole truth." Homeopathy gained prominence, he asserted, because of the inadequacy of heroic medicine. Wood quite correctly described Benjamin Rush as the epitome of the excesses of early American orthodoxy. In February and March of 1781, Rush was reported to have cured a Methodist minister of consumption by removing 8 pints of blood in a six-week period. In another case, the Philadelphian bled his patient 85 times in six months. Wood joked that it was a wonder "that enough of our forefathers survived the physicians of their day to give origin to the nation of the present." He went on to credit homeopathy with fostering a great revolution in orthodox medicine. The influence of the new school, he explained, did not result from any "truth contained in the theories of the German dreamer." Rather, it was because of the fact that the high dilution was safer than venesection and calomel. Wood insisted that but for homeopathy, the modern physician might still have been letting blood with reckless abandon, applying leeches, and administering massive doses of calomel. Perhaps the most significant revolution, however, was the one within homeopathy. Wood noted that few modern homeopaths followed the Hahnemannian pathways. The advanced homeopathic practitioner, he said, no longer was an uneducated quack. It was perfectly legiti-

[39] *North American Journal of Homeopathy*, 2d ser., 15 (November 1884): 286–88.

[40] C. A. Devenport, "Consultation and Affiliation with Homeopaths," *Michigan Medical News* 4 (December 24, 1881): 374–75.

mate, then, to consult with those men of science who continued to call themselves homeopaths.[41]

Other members of the traditionally conservative Philadelphia medical profession began to accept the homeopath as a well-trained physician. In 1889 Dr. Edward Jackson, professor of ophthalmology at the Philadelphia Polyclinic, read a paper on modern sectarianism to the county medical society. He declared that the curriculum of Hahnemann Medical College was not at all dogmatic. The students at this and other homeopathic colleges studied orthodox textbooks, such as Gray's *Anatomy* and Dalton's *Physiology*. Homeopathic teachings were restricted to *materia medica* and therapeutics. Jackson argued that since its graduates had learned the best of allopathic medicine, the college should be considered a "regular" school and its products, "regular" graduates. He declared that there was no reason to exclude anyone whose "conscientious convictions" led him away from the accepted practices.[42]

Dr. Solomon Solis-Cohen, professor of clinical medicine at the Polyclinic, commented upon Jackson's paper. He agreed that there were homeopaths who accepted scientific teachings in anatomy, physiology, surgery, and other nonsectarian fields. But he insisted that before being admitted to the counsels of orthodoxy they must abandon their homeopathic name. Since the term "homeopath" was a trademark, if they really were not practitioners of homeopathy, they were frauds who were using their label to attract unwitting patients. Only the dogmatic followers of Hahnemann, he said, should continue to be known as homeopaths. As the liberals were "regular" physicians in every way, and since they were willing to objectively test new theories, Solis-Cohen argued, they should be welcomed into the profession, but not as homeopaths.[43]

Although there was a notable change in the allopathic attitude toward homeopathy, much of the bitterness of the past remained. Some allopaths could not believe that homeopaths had modified their practice. In 1882 Alonzo B. Palmer, a center of attention in the Ann Arbor imbroglio, described "The Fallacies of Homeopathy." He declared that by definition, homeopaths could only dispense drugs on the basis of the law of similars.

[41] H. C. Wood, "The Medical Profession, the Medical Sects, and the Law," *New Englander* 51 (August 1889): 118–34.

[42] Edward Jackson, "Against Sectarianism in Medicine," *Medical News* 55 (October 19, 1889): 425–27.

[43] Solomon Solis-Cohen, "An Ethical Question," *Medical News* 55 (October 19, 1889): 427–35.

That meant, according to Palmer, that homeopaths could never consent to employ orthodox remedies.[44] Palmer and his followers, however, were thinking in terms of the homeopathy of the 1840's. By 1880 the majority of America's homeopaths were dispensing allopathic remedies in nonhomeopathic doses, along with the traditional homeopathic treatments. They wanted to consult with their orthodox colleagues and rejoin allopathic society.

[44] A. B. Palmer, "The Fallacies of Homeopathy," *North American Review* 134 (March 1882): 293–314.

IX

THE NEW CODE
AND ITS AFTERMATH

DURING THE EARLY 1880's, American physicians were quicker in facing the realities of the consultation problem than were their British counterparts. In England the most highly publicized dispute revolved around the fatal illness of Benjamin Disraeli, Lord Beaconsfield. When Joseph Kidd, a noted homeopath, was unable to cure the minister's severe attack of gout and bronchitis, Queen Victoria persuaded the doctor to ask Sir William Jenner for his assistance. Jenner, one of the foremost British physicians, placed his professional ethics before patriotism, and refused to consult with an irregular. Dr. Richard Quain, a top-flight surgeon, was next to be summoned. Willing to comply with the Queen's request, but at the same time wishing to be safe from professional attack, Quain sought the advice of Sir George Burrows, the former president of the College of Physicians and one of England's most highly respected practitioners. They decided to ask if Kidd was handling the case homeopathically. When Kidd's reply that he always treated "scientifically" did not satisfy them, he was asked to guarantee that "every direction and prescription of yours will be faithfully carried out by me [Kidd]," and being reassured on this point, Quain went to see Disraeli.[1]

On April 11, 1881, Quain found himself a center of controversy. At a session of the College of Physicians, he was denounced for having consulted with a homeopath. Two days earlier the *Lancet*, London's leading medical journal, had editorially condemned his violation of "a fundamental princi-

---

[1] *Medical Tribune* 3 (May 1881): 227–29; *New York Medical Eclectic* 8 (April 1881): 132–35.

ple of professional conduct." [2] Kidd hoped to protect Quain from further attack by explaining the situation. He asserted that he was no longer a homeopath. Almost five years earlier, he had resigned from several sectarian societies, and by 1881 he did not restrict himself to any one school of medical practice. Moreover, he noted that a "valuable life was at stake," and more important, "one precious to Her Most Gracious Majesty the Queen, and to many millions of her subjects." Kidd declared that Beaconsfield was so vital to the nation that professional differences should not have been allowed to prevent his recovery. [3]

While British physicians were still enforcing their version of the consultation clause, elements within the New York profession began to react to the changes which had occurred in allopathic and homeopathic medicine. A group within the Medical Society of the County of New York believed that the code of ethics had become an outmoded instrument which prevented physicians from following their consciences. Moreover, homeopaths were no longer "blinded" by theory; they had become eclectic in their practices. Perhaps most significant was the fact that homeopathy, having survived for over fifty years, was growing stronger. As early as the 1840's, in spite of the code, a number of physicians had consulted with homeopaths. The numbers of such consultations apparently increased as homeopathy grew more and more respectable; so by 1880 many physicians wanted it legalized. When many of the leading practitioners openly violated professional ethics, it was a strong indication that revision was required in the code of ethics.

Influenced by the members of the county society, on February 3, 1881, the Medical Society of the State of New York appointed a committee to study the A.M.A. code. On February 8, 1882, the committee reported its results, called by contemporaries the "new code." It differed from that of the national association in two respects. First, it not only prohibited all medical advertising, but it made it unethical for a physician to talk with a newspaper reporter. Then, and more significantly, it provided that fellows may consult with any "legally qualified practitioners of medicine. Emergencies may occur," it continued, "in which all restrictions should . . . yield to the demands of humanity." [4] Thus, the New York society began to dis-

---

[2] *Lancet* 1 (April 9, 1881): 587–88.

[3] *British Medical Journal* 1 (April 16, 1881): 620.

[4] *Transactions of the Medical Society of the State of New York, 1882* (Syracuse, 1882): 74–76; *New York Times,* February 14, 1882, p. 2, cols. 3–4.

cuss whether professional ethics should be brought into line with state laws which recognized the practice of homeopathy.

The most basic reason for the abandonment of the consultation clause was that a steadily increasing number of physicians had become convinced that homeopaths were well-educated men trying to minister to the sick. In addition, many allopaths argued that instead of destroying homeopathy, as was the intention of the orthodox actions, persecution had only strengthened it. Some advocates of the new code hoped that by sacrificing the A.M.A. code they eventually would effect a happy merger, in which homeopathy would disappear "as a special school of practice," with every physician adopting "what is valuable in the doctrines of Hahnemann, and forgetting distinctive names in professional fraternity." [5]

The defenders of the new code, usually younger physicians, argued that since homeopathy had been legalized in every state, it should receive professional recognition. Moreover, they declared that the old code was an infringement on the rights of "free American citizens," and especially a denial of the right to meet with any one, at any time, for any reason. Also, since the homeopathic and allopathic practices were similar, a restrictive code was an anachronism. The 1847 document was considered "old fogyism," a remnant of the days when morality had to be spelled out to the illiterate frontier doctors. Finally, the advocates of change insisted that in the interest of public health, a physician was obligated to give aid when asked, even if by a homeopath. [6]

Another source of opposition to the old code, always present but in the background, was the fear and hatred of organized labor and the industrial violence of the late 1870's. A number of physicians equated the old code with the "trades-union spirit" universally condemned by the middle and upper classes. [7]

The opponents of the new code generally were older men who recalled the dogmatic and obviously ridiculous homeopathy of the 1840's, refusing to admit that the homeopath had altered his practice in any way. Those who recognized that homeopathy had indeed evolved, insisted that homeopaths

---

[5] *New York Times*, February 14, 1882, p. 2, cols. 3–4. See the coverage of the new code controversy in Philip Van Ingen, *The New York Academy of Medicine: Its First Hundred Years* (New York, 1949), pp. 189–99, 204–5; and James J. Walsh, *History of the Medical Society of the State of New York* (New York, 1907), pp. 204–8.

[6] Frank Hastings Hamilton, *Conversations between Drs. Warren and Putnam on the Subject of Medical Ethics* (New York and London, 1884).

[7] *New York Daily Tribune*, February 5, 1883, p. 4, cols. 3–4.

were fraudulently using their trade-mark only to attract business. Moreover, the old code advocates noted that since the medical licensure laws did not raise educational standards, the profession had to assume responsibility for drawing the line between physician and charlatan. Is it our duty, they asked, to assist the charlatan in making his diagnosis?[8]

Further, they were quick to accuse the new-code advocates of having in mind only their own economic self-interest—of being specialists who hoped to add to their practice by allowing consultation with irregulars. That argument was partially true. The evidence indicates, however, that they were not primarily motivated by that consideration. There were simply too many general practitioners among the group for anyone to honestly attribute the new code to the rise of medical specialists. They were advocates of change because of their humanitarianism, along with their somewhat more realistic outlook.[9]

The bitterness of the conflict between the old and new code was evident at the 1882 meeting of the state medical society. After the committee reported the revised code, Dr. D. B. St. John Roosa, an ophthalmologist who taught both at the University of the City of New York and at the University of Vermont, took the floor. He was noted for a dominant personality, a "sonorous" voice, and a forceful expression, qualities which made him a formidable opponent. He declared that since every physician was fully capable of using discretion, there was no need for a code of ethics. He likened the code to a dictatorship, with the physicians as "children sitting at their mother's feet."[10]

Roosa's substitute for the code was a simple statement that the only ethical violations should be "acts unworthy [of] a physician and a gentleman." Although winning a majority, 40 to 38, Roosa's proposal lost for lack of the necessary two-thirds vote. Then Dr. Henry Piffard, who had helped to draft the new code, moved to adopt the committee report. By a vote of 52 to 18, the New York state medical society substituted the revised standard for that of the A.M.A.[11]

New York's leading newspapers were quick to editorialize upon the conflict in the profession. The *Daily Tribune* reported that "there is a good

---

[8] Hamilton, *Conversations*, passim.

[9] *New York Daily Tribune*, February 5, 1883, p. 4, cols. 3–4; *New York Times*, January 17, 1884, p. 1, col. 7.

[10] *Transactions of the Medical Society, State of New York, 1882*, pp. 26–28, 74–76.

[11] Ibid., pp. 48–50.

deal of sense" in the abandonment of the consultation clause.[12] On the other hand, the *Times* applauded the change in the consultation clause, but it bitterly condemned the section of the new code which prohibited advertising and which denied the right of doctors to give information to reporters. The editorial insisted that the new code meant the end of free speech in the profession, but it did not mention that it also would end a lucrative source of revenue for a great many magazines and newspapers.[13]

The new code, however, was not so eagerly accepted by the profession. In fact, twelve of the fourteen state medical associations which met prior to the 1882 A.M.A. convention passed "very strong resolutions" condemning their New York colleagues. In addition, orthodox journals were almost unanimous in their denunciation of the changes. The *Maryland Medical Journal*, for instance, said that "it will not elevate the standing of the regular profession, whilst it will give credit and respectability to quackery and professional irregularity." The *Louisville Medical News* expressed a hope that the "ill-advised" action would be reconsidered. The *Detroit Lancet* added its assertion that "however the commercial spirit may dominate the profession of the State of New York, it will not dominate every other state." The *Ohio Medical Journal* expressed what must have been the last word when it exclaimed: "Fifty-two doctors at Albany, reckless of honor, but greedy for gold, undertook to sell out the regular profession, but only succeeded in selling themselves, and very cheap at that."[14]

On June 7, 1882 the American Medical Association convened at St. Paul, amid the almost complete condemnation of the new code. The judicial council was asked to rule on the seating of the New York delegation, which had been challenged on the basis of its opposition to the old code. The council decided that by announcing a revised code, the state society had forfeited its right to representation at national conventions. When the ruling was adopted, "great applause" was reported in the hall.[15]

The action of the A.M.A. was more than another attack upon those wishing to recognize homeopathy. It was closely related to the differences between physicians of the east and those of the other sections of the country. Although the seaboard states had a relatively ineffective licensure system, the western and southern states generally had none at all. Indeed, condi-

---

[12] *New York Daily Tribune*, February 16, 1882, p. 4, col. 5.

[13] *New York Times*, February 19, 1882, p. 8, col. 6.

[14] All cited in *New England Medical Gazette* 17 (June 1882): 165–68.

[15] *Transactions of the A.M.A.* 33 (Philadelphia, 1882): 33; *New York Times*, June 8, 1882, p. 5, col. 6.

tions in the west were so dismal that the "businessmen" who operated diploma mills recommended that their "graduates" settle in the west.[16] The western physician, then, must have felt a greater need for ethical considerations than did the practitioners on the east coast. Moreover, western homeopathic colleges were far inferior to those established earlier in Pennsylvania, New York, and Massachusetts. The irregular profession of the relatively unsettled areas was then clearly inferior to that of the east. Thus, the New York society was thinking in terms of consulting with well-qualified homeopaths, while the western and southern allopaths could not think of having any professional relations with such "impostors." Since the convention was held in the midwest, the eastern delegations were limited, while the western states were over-represented. A number of physicians who might have defended the actions of the New Yorkers were notably missing from the 1882 meeting. The result was that the western allopaths pushed through a condemnation of the empire state society.

The *New York Times* was fast to condemn the A.M.A. for having expelled the New York delegates, especially since it seemed apparent that the old code was hopelessly inadequate. The editorial asserted that by its actions, the national association had declared that the patient must die rather than be saved through an "unethical" consultation. The New York doctors, it continued, could survive quite well without the A.M.A. and the doctors from "Oshkosh and Okolona." "Pity the unfortunate patients who are in the hands of men who think that their own narrow-minded prejudices should never yield to humanity."[17]

The next year the *Times* declared that according to the old code, "A person who employs a homeopathic physician is worthy of death." The editor jokingly suggested that the difficulty might be settled by passing a law making it a felony "for any person willfully and knowingly to employ a homeopathist." The penalty, he said, should not be immediate death, but rather a term in the state prison, "together with treatment by 'regular' physicians."[18]

Besides newspapers, leading magazines began to take stands in favor of the new code. E. L. Godkin, the editor of the *Nation*, for instance, editorialized on "The Medical War." He applauded the humane physicians who

[16] Martin Kaufman, "American Medical Diploma Mills," *Bulletin of the Tulane Medical Faculty* 26 (February 1967): 56.

[17] *New York Times,* June 9, 1882, p. 4, cols. 5–6. See also the comments on newspaper opinion in *Michigan Medical News* 5 (June 26, 1882): 177–78.

[18] *New York Times*, May 3, 1883, p. 4, col. 5.

were willing to consult with irregulars in order to benefit humanity. Even if the homeopaths were "absolute and recognized impostors," he declared, it would not be reason enough to refuse to assist one of their patients. Godkin said that the situation reminded him of the Irish priest who always complained about his congregation, "whose evil ways he was unable to restrain even by occasional horsewhipping." When asked whether he had ever tried the Gospel on his flock, the good father replied indignantly that "he was not going to waste good Gospel on the likes of 'em." [19]

Although the New Yorkers were more forward looking than their more conservative colleagues, their position was basically inconsistent. The New York society could hardly expect to abandon a cherished and sacred document, the old code, and remain affiliated with the American Medical Association. Acceptance of the code of ethics had not only been the major prerequisite for admission to the national fraternity, but many of its constituent societies had expelled members for having violated the code. Any society which rejected tradition had in effect written itself out of the profession. Yet the New Yorkers thought that they could revise the code and remain within organized medicine.

When some members realized that they had ostracized themselves, they sought to remedy the situation by repealing the new code. In 1883, at the annual meeting of the state society, Brooklyn's Dr. Edward R. Squibb, a physician who was noted for his pharmaceutical business, introduced a series of resolutions demanding that the society return to the A.M.A. code of ethics. Dr. Roosa entered the debate, declaring that unlike many of his colleagues, he did not fear the word "revolutionary," which the opponents of the new code were using to discredit innovation. "All the advances in the world," he said, "have been made by revolutions." "We claim for ourselves, not the privilege of 'affiliating with quacks,' but of giving our advice wherever it is asked for, whether by Homeopath or Eclectic, Zulu or Modoc." After the extremely vocal discussion, the new-code advocates narrowly defeated their opponents, 105 to 95, retaining the revised version of the code of ethics and preventing the reunification of the profession.[20]

Because of the importance of the topic at hand, the profession turned out en masse for the monthly meetings of almost every major New York medical organization. Every physician seemed to want to be present for every crucial vote on any segment of the new-code controversy. Unfortunately

[19] *Nation* 36 (April 26, 1883): 357.
[20] *Transactions of the Medical Society, State of New York, 1883*, pp. 25–27, 35–36, 73.

for many practitioners, being available for every vote meant having to sit through papers on such items as puerperal septicemia and "boiler maker's deafness." Then, on January 29, 1883, some excitement developed. Roosa, who had become the leader of the fight to revise the code, proposed that the county medical society announce its acceptance of the new code. After a typically bitter debate, and after Dr. Austin Flint, one of the most distinguished physicians of his time, condemned the new code, Roosa's resolution was adopted by a vote of 135 to 43.[21]

Now that the county society had sided with the liberal faction, the ever-conservative New York Academy of Medicine moved into the arena. On April 19, through careful planning, the old-code advocates managed to pack the hall. Austin Flint, Jr., a leading physiologist who was following in his father's footsteps in more ways than one, proposed that the Academy adopt the old code. He also proposed that any one who could not follow every provision of the A.M.A. ethical standard should not be admitted to fellowship. Roosa added to the electrified atmosphere when he declared that Flint's resolution was part of a grand plot; "a secret society, trying to destroy the Academy, had ordered its members to be present." After Roosa was hooted down with a chorus of "jeers and derisive laughter," the old-code faction voted, 58 to 25, to retain the 1847 document, and to admit no more "traitors."

At that point in the proceedings, Fordyce Barker, a gynecologist who was president of the Academy, R. F. Weir, the vice president, and W. F. Cushman, the treasurer, joined Roosa in submitting their resignations. Bitterness was rife; an old-code man, Dr. Samuel S. Purple, was reported to have exclaimed: "I hope the gentlemen have paid their dues."[22] Two days later, the *New York Herald* reported that Barker told a reporter: "It was a disgraceful, abominable trick, and only fit to be undertaken by a low ward politician. In doing this, [Flint] pulled down his venerable father from a pinnacle that was beautiful and lovely and dragged him in the mud."[23]

In 1883 the American Medical Association made compromise almost impossible and turned the difficulty into a national problem. First, every delegate to the Cleveland convention was asked to sign a pledge of allegiance to the old code of ethics. That meant that every physician had to choose between the two codes, and selection of the new code meant voluntary exile

[21] *New York Times*, January 30, 1883, p. 5, col. 4.
[22] *New York Medical Journal* 37 (April 28, 1883): 462–63; *New York Times*, April 21, 1883, p. 2, col. 3.
[23] *New York Medical Journal* 37 (May 5, 1883): 500.

from the ranks of orthodoxy. Then, a proposal was tabled which might have prevented a schism. That resolution would have authorized the formation of a committee to examine the old code and revise it to meet the needs of the day. Unfortunately, when it was tabled by the delegates, the A.M.A. had turned its back upon reunification.[24]

On October 15, 1883, the advocates of the old code met to map out strategy in advance of the upcoming session of the New York Academy of Medicine. Three days later, 215 members attended the monthly meeting, a far cry from the 50 who normally found time to add to their scientific knowledge and fraternize with their old friends. The ethical problem was the only item under discussion at that meeting. Fordyce Barker, whose resignation had not been acted upon, presented a series of amendments to abolish the by-law which accepted the A.M.A. code as that of the Academy. Although it had a majority, by 121 to 92, the proposal failed to receive the necessary three-fourths vote. Then the new-code men suggested that the resolution of April 19 be rescinded. As noted earlier, that proposal prevented the admittance of any one opposed to the old code. Although they had been unable to repeal the by-law, the April action was annulled.[25]

Later that month, on October 22, the battle shifted to the county medical society, which had initiated the entire problem in 1880. That meeting was a crucial one, as it was to include the annual election of officers. The elections were usually noncontroversial. Normally, a list of candidates was prepared in advance, with one physician for each vacancy. In 1883 the new-code advocates nominated a slate, while the old coders proposed their own candidates. Legally, but rather unethically, the liberals brought eighty new members, who were admitted and then allowed to cast their ballots for the new code. The eighty votes, however, were unnecessary. The old-code men were defeated by about 380 to 215 for every office.[26]

Toward the end of 1883, the advocates of the old code established the "Central Organization of the New-York State Medical Association to Uphold the National Code of Ethics." They sent questionnaires to 5,219 physicians, and 65 per cent of those who responded were in favor of the A.M.A. code of ethics. On the basis of their discovery that the majority of the New York profession remained loyal to the old code, the leading con-

---

[24] *Journal of the American Medical Association* 1 (July 14, 1883): 9; *New York Daily Tribune*, June 6, 1883, p. 1, col. 3.

[25] *New York Daily Tribune*, October 19, 1883, p. 5, cols. 2-3; *New York Medical Journal* 38 (October 27, 1883): 467.

[26] *New York Times*, October 23, 1883, p. 5, col. 2.

servatives wanted to establish a New York state medical association which would accept the 1847 ethical standard and send delegates to the national conventions.

The old-code faction called a meeting on February 4, 1884, the day before the state society was to vote once again on a proposal to rescind the new code. The minutes of that gathering indicate that the conservatives were convinced that the new code was pushed through by an unscrupulous minority which acted in accordance with a "pre-arranged plan." They claimed that a small percentage had taken actions which severed all ties with the national profession, contrary to the wishes of the majority. Moreover, the old coders were aghast at having to abandon "the most sacred traditions of the profession." Austin Flint, Jr., declared that "no physician can be true to his calling and manhood and yet be willing to meet as a professional brother a charlatan or one who practices medicine with a dishonest designation." [27]

Furthermore, the old-code faction was certain that the liberals were taking illegal and unparliamentary steps, such as the packing of the Academy with eighty new members. Also the fact that more than a majority was required to recall the old code meant that the minority was hiding "under the shield" of a two-thirds vote, preventing the will of the majority. After all the discussion at the planning session, the conservatives decided that if the state society failed to restore the A.M.A. document, they would reconvene and formally establish the New York State Medical Association. [28] The following day, in the face of threatened secession, by a vote of 124 to 105, the state society once again refused to return to the old code, and the Association was organized on February 6. [29]

In 1885 the new code threatened to destroy the Ninth International Medical Congress. During the eighth congress, at Copenhagen, the eight Americans in attendance were invited to host the next convention. Immediately accepting the honor, the delegates took it upon themselves to decide upon the composition of the committees in the various specialties. Then they reported to the A.M.A. convention at New Orleans that the Congress would be held in Washington, D.C., and they read the names of the various participants.

The southern and western delegates were outraged to learn that the op-

[27] *Transactions of the New York State Medical Association* 1 (New York, 1885): 504–14.
[28] Ibid., pp. 514–18.
[29] *Transactions of the Medical Society, State of New York, 1884,* pp. 40–45.

ponents of the code were named to positions on the committees. They demanded that, regardless of international reputations, no new-code men should be allowed to remain as honorary vice presidents. In addition, the westerners and southerners insisted that there be a more equitable geographical distribution of honors. Since most of the prominent physicians were concentrated in New York City, Philadelphia, and Boston, the list of honors appeared to some practitioners to be a who's who of the northeast and of the new-code advocates. The old-code faction demanded that more doctors from their sections be added to the committees.[30]

The A.M.A. decided that only those physicians who accepted the code of ethics could serve on any committee of the International Congress. This eliminated the new-code men, which included such eminent physicians as Dr. Abraham Jacobi, the pediatrician who had spent from 1851 to 1853 in Prussian prisons for his political activities, and who had demonstrated his liberalism by marrying a pioneering lady doctor, Mary Putnam. Other New Yorkers who were summarily dismissed from positions in the Congress were Roosa and Barker. Among the Bostonians expelled were Henry I. Bowditch and Francis Minot, the latter a prominent member of the Harvard medical faculty. As news of the A.M.A. action spread across the nation, physicians who were appointed to the committees began to announce that they could not serve without such leading men as Jacobi and Bowditch, and others refused to replace physicians who had been expelled for their opinions.[31] It began to look as if the first international recognition of American medicine might be lost.

Bowditch assumed the leadership of the forces opposed to both the A.M.A. and its outmoded ethical code. As a result of his willingness to take a stand on what he considered a moral issue, the Association took punitive action. Bowditch, who had been secretary in 1847, vice president in 1863, and president in 1877, found his name removed from the "hallowed" list of former presidents of the A.M.A. Alfred Stillé, the Philadelphian, wrote to inform him that in his opinion the A.M.A. "has sunk steadily to lower levels & ceased to inspire the least respect. Of all the personal affronts it has given," he said, "the grossest was its dropping your name from the list of Presidents."[32]

By October of 1885 the A.M.A. leadership recognized that it had alien-

[30] *New York Medical Journal* 42 (July 11, 1885): 44–45.
[31] Ibid.
[32] Stillé to Bowditch, July 24, 1885, MS in Bowditch monographs, folder 10 D, Countway Library, Harvard University.

ated so many top-flight physicians that the International Congress would practically be devoid of American representatives of high scientific accomplishment. At that point, N. S. Davis wrote to inform Bowditch that he had unanimously been elected vice president of the Congress, indicating that the old-code advocates had withdrawn from their earlier stand. To prevent further strife, Davis urged Bowditch to forget the past and assume his position. Bowditch, who during the Civil War had been so vigorous in his espousal of abolitionism that he was ostracized from Boston society, angrily replied that he absolutely refused to accept so late an apology.[33]

Bowditch then wrote to ask Surgeon-General John S. Billings if he would start a debate on the need for a new code of ethics at the forthcoming meeting of the A.M.A. Billings replied to the effect that he recognized that Bowditch was correct on the code, and unlike others, able to take a stand without fearing the consequences. "I believe that attempts to make such a change will simply increase bitterness of feeling," the Surgeon-General wrote, "and increase the disgrace of the profession in the eyes of the non-medical public." He begged Bowditch not to force him to make a stand or an official statement. Opposition by the A.M.A. could result in the loss of his valued position. "Leave me in peace and as much obscurity as possible," he entreated. The Library of Medicine, Johns Hopkins, and the Surgeon-General's Catalogue were all more important to Billings, and to medicine, than either the composition of the International Medical Congress or the need for a new code of ethics. Billings concluded by urging Bowditch to rest upon his laurels.[34]

Bowditch, however, was unable to remain silent. On June 10, 1886, he read a most provocative paper at the 75th anniversary meeting of the Rhode Island Medical Society. It later was published, entitled *The Past, Present, and Future Treatment of Homeopathy, Eclecticism, and Kindred Delusions*. He began by declaring that the code of ethics had driven American doctors "to acts of intolerance reminding one of Mediaeval clerical tyranny." He asserted that homeopathy and eclecticism "are the legitimate offsprings of the absurdities of the Medical Profession itself. The arrant nonsense exhibited by our fathers in the so-called 'good old times' of our art begat these two Infinitesimal and Eclectic Idiots, as some of you may call them."[35]

---

[33] Davis to Bowditch, Chicago, October 8, 1885; Bowditch to Davis, October 12, 1885, MSS in Bowditch monographs, folder 11.

[34] Billings to Bowditch, Washington, D.C., October 25, 1885, MS in Bowditch monographs, folder 11 O.

[35] Henry I. Bowditch, *The Past, Present, and Future Treatment of Homeopathy, Eclecticism and Kindred Delusions* (Boston, 1887), pp. 5–7.

For those who could not understand how any physician could abandon orthodox medicine, Bowditch graphically illustrated his case. He described the results of calomel, "the poor wretch lying on one side for perhaps days unable to swallow even liquids without torture and with his tongue swollen to three or four times its usual size, protruded far beyond the lips, intensely sore, while from its tip a constant string of adhesive and stinking mucus was discharging into a spittoon below it!" It was no wonder, he said, that the "stalwart irregular," Thomson, exclaimed: "All this is too horrible to be tolerated. Come, come to me, ye afflicted ones! I use only God's holy herbs in the treatments of your ailments."[36]

The Boston physician first urged the allopaths to "follow the lead of New York" and consult with any legally registered practitioners. Then, those sectarians who stopped calling themselves by an exclusive name should be admitted into professional society. Third, he insisted that his colleagues urge the A.M.A. to admit delegates from the Medical Society of the State of New York. Finally, Bowditch demanded that the national association rescind its order that every member annually swear to uphold the code of ethics.[37]

Dr. Alexander Y. P. Garnett, a former Confederate surgeon who had settled in Washington, D.C., published a short pamphlet refuting Bowditch. The copy on file in the Bowditch papers at the Countway Medical Library includes a number of marginal notes written by Bowditch, in his almost illegible scrawl. Taken together, one can easily understand the different sides to the dispute. Garnett began his defense of the A.M.A. by asserting that the code of ethics had had a profound influence for thirty-five years. He said that it had harmonized physicians into a brotherhood, promoting "love of profession, personal honor, integrity, and self respect." Prior to the acceptance of the code in 1847, he said that there was "fierce internecine strife," even affecting the choice of delegates from Massachusetts. To that charge, Bowditch replied in the margin: "Purely imaginary," and "do not remember."[38]

On this point, however, Garnett was correct. In 1846 "one of the most respectable medical societies" of Boston tabled a proposal to "appoint a committee to *enquire into the Expediency* of Sending delegates" to the first national convention. Alfred Stillé wrote at the time that the action would

[36] Ibid., pp. 10–11.
[37] Ibid., pp. 11–16.
[38] *Letter of A. Y. P. Garnett, M.D., in reply to Henry I. Bowditch, November, 1887* (Washington, D.C., 1887), p. 2. All citations to this short pamphlet are to the annotated copy in the Bowditch Papers, Countway Library.

reinforce the "vulgar prejudice that New Englanders are narrow-minded and Selfish, wanting in those more generous impulses which urge a man to risk something of their own comfort for the sake of the general good." "Surely," he said, "our Boston friends must be under some temporary hallucination." [39]

Garnett continued to note that in 1884, the A.M.A. was so liberal and compromising that it had appointed a five-man committee to "review and prepare an authorized construction of its code of ethics." Bowditch scribbled: "Instead of having a committee *revise* the Code." Moreover, this committee included such conservatives as Austin Flint and N. S. Davis, and they intended to explain the provisions of the code, "treating the members in fact like little children and incapable of judging for themselves of the *actual operations* of the Code." [40]

Although Garnett emphasized professional harmony and brotherhood, he insisted that there was "widespread demoralization and decadence of personal integrity and honor." He said that conditions were so bad that it was necessary to check on "disreputable and dishonest modes and methods." Bowditch declared in response that honorable men needed no moral code, while Garnett had been convinced that man was basically immoral, needing laws to guide his conduct. Bowditch scratched in the pamphlet: "Does Dr. Garnett mean to say that the majority of medical men are devils incarnate?" Garnett answered a few pages later. He said that "in the race between virtue and vice," "the fleet-footed and ubiquitous Satan has far outstripped the tardy Bourbons of Christ, and that at this advanced period of so-called moral ideas men are only restrained from wrong-doing by the apprehension of some punitive consequences to themselves." [41]

One must remember that Garnett was writing in an age which had witnessed widespread corruption during Reconstruction, which had uncovered the graft of the Tweed Ring, which had discovered payoffs and kickbacks in the Credit Mobilier scandals, and during which some "Robber Barons" were sweeping aside all ethical values in their quest for riches. It did indeed seem as if the "fleet-footed and ubiquitous Satan" were victorious, although there was not much reason to condemn educated physicians.

Garnett continued to declare that if only for self-preservation, the A.M.A. had to require a signed pledge by its members, "in order to distinguish friend from foe." It could not be expected to "admit into its

[39] Alfred Stillé to Jonathan Watson, Philadelphia, January 30, 1847, MS in Gratz collection, Historical Society of Pennsylvania.

[40] *Letter of A. Y. P. Garnett*, p. 3.

[41] Ibid., p. 5.

councils a Trojan horse filled with declared enemies." Bowditch happily scribbled in the margin: "Delightful brotherhood."[42]

As far as Bowditch was concerned, the major issue was the attempt of the A.M.A. to control the views of its membership. He declared that he and his colleagues were capable of distinguishing right from wrong. On the other hand, Garnett had less faith in the morality of the average physician.

Interestingly, although the conservatives were fighting to prevent the recognition of homeopathy, Bowditch himself did not want to consult with irregulars. In 1885 he wrote in the draft of an address that he had never consulted with any doctor "who believes in Infinitesimals." During the past year, he had met with an eclectic, and he found that gentleman "equal in acquirements to any regular physician."[43] And, in his correspondence on whether a *"Homeopathic Surgeon!"* should be allowed to read books at the medical library, Bowditch ridiculed homeopathy for its inconsistencies and for its emphasis upon high dilutions. He respected all opinions, however, and he was willing to assist in the treatment of any patient, whether aiding a homeopath or a physician who was the epitome of orthodoxy.[44]

The homeopathic reaction to the new-code controversy was one of the more interesting aspects of the entire situation. They should have been encouraged and pleased at the spirit of liberality exhibited by the new-code advocates. In actuality, however, their reaction was quite the opposite. In editorializing on the New York affair, the *Hahnemannian Monthly* exclaimed: "it is the old invitation of the spider to the fly." "Will you walk into my parlor," the allopaths were saying, ready to destroy homeopathy by chicanery and diplomacy now that persecution had so obviously failed. The editor predicted that the next step would be for the orthodox profession to accept homeopaths who were willing to renounce their heritage. In a later issue, the same editor exclaimed that the new code "would rob us of our individuality, despoil us of our precious laurels, steal our therapeutic weapons, and then cast us into oblivion."[45]

In June of 1882 the *New England Medical Gazette*, another leading

---

[42] Ibid., p. 6.

[43] Henry I. Bowditch, "Codes of Medical Ethics: Their Evil Influence when interpreted by Bigoted Partisanship of Societies or Individuals," MS in Bowditch Papers.

[44] Henry I. Bowditch, Correspondence with Dr. E. H. Bradford on allowing a *"Homeopathic Surgeon!"* to read books at our medical library. The absurdity of their original expulsion from the Massachusetts Medical Society, 1889, MS in Bowditch Papers.

[45] *Hahnemannian Monthly* 17 (March 1882): 176–81; 17 (October 1882): 623–26.

homeopathic publication, trying to explain the sudden change of heart, agreed with the critics who argued that persecution had ceased because it had been proved ineffectual. Then the editor noted that others had suggested that the new code had been formulated by the specialists who had most to gain from consultation. If that were the case, the New York movement was devoid of humanitarianism; it was merely a "bid for increased patronage." He concluded by declaring that although allopathic medicine and the advocates of the new code would benefit from the change, liberal men "first prompted this important step,—men who found the old restrictions upon individual choice in matters of professional conduct both unbearable and unwarrantable in the light of modern progress." Let us simply "recognize the fact that some liberal men in the old school accord to us an honest purpose, and insist upon freedom to both give and receive assistance in the great work of our common profession." [46]

Despite the changes which had occurred in homeopathy as well as in allopathic medicine, and regardless of the changing attitude as exemplified in the new-code controversy, the orthodox profession still had a long way to go before it could accept the homeopath as a brother. In 1882 the Massachusetts Medical Society charged Dr. Frederick F. Moore, of New York, with having aided and abetted an irregular practitioner. His defense counsel, Dr. David Hunt, became so wrapped up in his oratory that he argued that the consultation clause was such a "dead letter" that he was quite willing to admit that he had consulted with irregulars, as had many other prominent physicians. Hunt was unable to prevent the expulsion of Moore, and three weeks later he was to argue his own case. Happily for Hunt, the only damaging evidence was his own "confession." When Drs. Oliver Wendell Holmes and Henry I. Bowditch, among others, testified to Hunt's good character and professional accomplishments, the case was dropped. [47]

Early in the 1880's, however, the allopaths did begin to waver in their attitude toward homeopathy, and later in that decade real changes were to take place, changes that eventually threatened to destroy homeopathy by submerging it within the orthodox profession.

[46] *New England Medical Gazette* 17 (May 1882): 129–31.
[47] Massachusetts Medical Society, Records of Boards of Trial since 1882, MS in possession of the Society.

X

REORGANIZATION AND REUNIFICATION

DURING THE LAST THREE DECADES of the nineteenth century, the continuing conflict between homeopathy and orthodoxy was intensified by the drive to improve the state medical licensure laws. The allopathic profession sought to enact legislation providing for the examination of all applicants by a board of physicians acceptable to the A.M.A., or at least a board with an orthodox majority. At first, most homeopaths thought that a unified examining board would be the first step toward the elimination of their system. They were convinced, not without justification, that the traditionally intolerant allopaths would never grant licenses to irregular practitioners and that the formation of a unified examining board would allow the enemy to serve as judge and executioner.

As time passed, other factors operated to change the attitude of both allopath and homeopath. For instance, physicians of each sect became convinced that in order to ensure an adequate system of medical care, incompetent practitioners had to be driven out of business. This recognition was reinforced when it became known that, in addition to the graduates of the many inferior proprietary schools, thousands of totally unprepared "doctors" were annually being turned loose upon an unsuspecting public by a number of diploma mills. Medical licensure laws were becoming more necessary than ever before.

A second factor was the growth of a number of smaller sects, each of which demanded their "constitutional right" to practice upon an unwitting public. Foremost among the minor practitioners were the osteopaths, the followers of Andrew T. Still, who claimed that the proper placement of bones was the key to health. Next were the chiropractors, led by Daniel D. Palmer, who emphasized the position of the spine. Finally came the Christian Scientists, headed by Mary Baker Eddy. In order to protect themselves from unethical competition and society from untrained "physicians," allopaths and homeopaths were forced to unite behind legislation which would guarantee their own existence, but would eliminate the minor sects.

As noted earlier, the development of Jacksonian democracy in the 1830's and 1840's combined with several other factors to bring about the repeal of America's early medical license laws. In almost every state, anyone who considered himself competent could call himself "Doctor," hang out a shingle, and open an office. During the 1870's many states reacted to the influx of quack and charlatan by passing restrictive statutes. Since the new laws usually accepted a medical diploma as evidence of qualification, they provided simply for registration of practitioners, encouraging unscrupulous operators to set up printing presses and to sell diplomas to those who wanted to become physicians. In 1880 and 1881, when the existence of diploma mills was widely publicized, the respectable practitioners came to recognize that more effective legislation was needed.[1]

The diploma salesmen were among the most unethical businessmen of the notoriously corrupt "Gilded Age." The most infamous of such scoundrels, John Buchanan, not only was known to have granted degrees to two-year-old children, whose parents could afford the fee, but he issued others after a two-day course of study intended to give some semblance of legitimacy. When he finally was arrested after having tried to escape to Canada, Buchanan admitted to having sold 60,000 diplomas at prices from $10 to $200. Men like Buchanan openly advertised and offered a selection of "colleges" to the prospective purchaser. One concern even ran a going-out-of-business sale, disposing of their entire stock of diplomas at bargain basement prices.[2]

Obviously, the possession of a diploma was no guarantee of proficiency, especially when so often the only prerequisite was the ability to pay. The publicity given to the diploma mill scandals brought a demand for revision of the licensure laws. In 1880 the Massachusetts legislature began to debate a bill to protect society from the unqualified practitioner. It provided for the formation of a nine-man board, composed of five or six allopaths, one

---

[1] John H. Rauch, "Address in State Medicine," *Journal of the A.M.A.* 6 (June 12, 1886): 645–52; see also Richard H. Shryock, *Medical Licensing in America, 1650–1965* (Baltimore, 1967), chapter II.

[2] Martin Kaufman, "American Medical Diploma Mills," *Bulletin of the Tulane Medical Faculty* 26 (February 1967): 53–57.

or two homeopaths, one eclectic, and one dentist. Under this board, every applicant for a license would have been required to pass an examination and demonstrate proficiency in the various fields of medical science. Drs. Herbert C. Clapp, David Thayer, I. T. Talbot, Conrad Wesselhoeft, and H. E. Spalding, all prominent homeopaths, joined with many allopaths in announcing their support of the proposal.[3]

Despite the desperate need for the bill and the backing of many leading allopaths and homeopaths, passage was far from automatic. A great many persons would be directly affected, and, according to one journal, the "vampires who would inevitably be driven out of the State" flocked to defend their interests. Present at the legislative hearings were "medical blacklegs of all kinds; deceitful clairvoyants, long-haired spiritualists, necromancers, wizards, witches, seers, magnetic healers, pain charmers, big Indian and negro doctors," and abortionists. Many of these were the unethical "harpies who excite the fears and prey on the 'indiscretions' of the young of both sexes, who treat venereal diseases with the utmost secrecy and despatch, who have good facilities for providing comfortable board for females suffering from any irregularity or obstruction, who sell pills which they are very particular to caution women when pregnant against using." Most of the opponents of the bill reportedly had a "coarse, animal, degraded look, enough to send a chill through a person of fine sensibilities."[4]

The proposal had the support of many groups of practitioners. Among those who were willing to endorse the bill were the members of the New England Society of Specialists. This organization consisted of men who had ruined their professional reputations by advertising and by promising to cure. It excluded the venereal disease specialists, who were considered to be at the bottom of the medical barrel. The Society announced that it would not oppose the bill if its present membership was licensed without having to undergo examination.[5]

The Massachusetts Medical Society also wanted "some kind of a law," but many of its members had qualms about any recognition of homeopathy. Although some allopaths insisted that orthodox physicians should have no dealings with irregulars, the proposed examining board would include homeopaths and eclectics. The more conservative physicians rejected any bill except one giving the A.M.A. complete control. The majority of the allopaths, however, realized that there were "worse evils" in the medical

---

[3] *New England Medical Gazette* 15 (February 1880): 35–36.
[4] Ibid. (March 1880): 65–66.
[5] Ibid., pp. 66–67.

community than the followers of Hahnemann. Most of the orthodox physicians, then, were willing to co-operate with homeopaths in order to eliminate quacks and pretenders, a category which not too long before had included homeopaths. A final allopathic faction was eager to consult with homeopaths, feeling that they were sincere and honest practitioners who had been unfairly treated in the past.[6]

The irregular profession maintained three distinct points of view. One group advocated a unified medical board, depending upon the honesty and good will of the allopathic majority. Another group demanded equal representation. They insisted that the licensing agency include three allopaths, three homeopaths, and three eclectics, a demand which disregarded the fact that in terms of numbers the orthodox practitioners were a distinct majority. There were roughly ten allopaths for every homeopath, and there were even fewer eclectics. This group argued that a board dominated by allopaths was not likely to do justice to the claims of homeopaths and eclectics. The third irregular faction opposed the formation of any medical examining board. "Let the fittest survive," they exclaimed, resting their fate upon the belief in the tenets of conservative social Darwinism.[7]

After four years of bitter fighting, the bill became law. In 1884 allopaths, homeopaths, and eclectics were appointed to the Massachusetts Medical Examining Board, with the orthodox profession holding the balance of power. The result was that the quacks who had been licensed out of Canada and later driven out of New Hampshire and Vermont, were now forced out of Massachusetts and sent on to greener pastures in the West.[8]

In trying to enact licensure laws, New York and the other states encountered the same divisions in the medical profession. In 1882 the *New York Medical Times*, a homeopathic journal edited by the ultra-liberal Dr. Egbert Guernsey, advocated a unified examining board. His ideas, however, were contrary to the ideas of the majority of the homeopaths, who favored separate boards in order to ensure that allopaths would not be given control over the licensure of irregulars. Guernsey, who continued to argue for one board, declared that it would help to "break down the sectarian and clannish feeling which now prevails."[9]

The *American Homeopath*, edited by the more reactionary George Winterburn, took an opposite stand. It insisted that no bill could "do justice

[6] Ibid.
[7] *New England Medical Gazette* 15 (March 1880): 67–70.
[8] Ibid.
[9] *New York Medical Times* 10 (April 1882): 20–21.

to the minority." "Equal representation, three separate boards, or nothing, is what we demand, preferably the last."[10] Winterburn later exclaimed: "Every man has the right to employ any other man to do any thing for him, whether it be to take care of his horse or his health." "We would not submit to legislature enactment compelling us to patronize John, the butcher, and Dick, the baker, and we see no reason why they should be compelled to have a doctor endorsed by government." With free competition, he said, the best physicians would thrive, while the weaker ones would fall by the wayside.[11]

In 1885 the American Institute of Homeopathy took an official stand against the "attempt of the A.M.A." to control licensure. It declared that under no circumstances should homeopaths let the allopaths decide their destiny. Despite the opposition of organized homeopathy, in 1889 Guernsey once again urged the formation of a single New York examining board, composed of five allopaths, three homeopaths, and one eclectic. Like many allopaths, Guernsey hoped to eradicate sectarianism by having every physician undergo an examination in anatomy, physiology, surgery, and the other medical fields.[12]

A great many homeopaths, however, were in no hurry to hand over the licensure system to their allopathic enemies. The Homeopathic Medical Society of the County of New York adopted a resolution stating that a single board, controlled by allopaths, would "bring about the obliteration of the homeopathic school." It called for every American homeopath to unite in "aggressive action," to frame a bill which would preserve homeopathic identity while eliminating incompetent physicians.[13]

Partly as a result of the popular revulsion against the allopathic intolerance and in part because of the upper class clientele of homeopathy, the irregulars held the balance of power in the New York State legislature. In order to suppress quackery, the orthodox physicians had to compromise by supporting a less stringent bill than they would have preferred. On September 1, 1891, New York's medical practice act went into effect, with three separate seven-man boards of examiners. The respective medical societies nominated the candidates for positions on the board, while the regents of the state university selected the examination questions. Therapeutics was

---

[10] *American Homeopath* 10 (January 1884): 26.
[11] Ibid. (March 1884): 86.
[12] *New England Medical Gazette* 20 (July 1885): 323–29; *North American Journal of Homeopathy*, 3d ser., 4 (April 1889): 50–51.
[13] *New York Times*, October 11, 1889, p. 4, col. 7; see also *Hahnemannian Monthly* 25 (February 1890): 86–92.

included on the test, but the questions were in harmony with the tenets of the school selected by the applicant.[14]

The first few years of licensure indicated that neither group had much to fear. Each sect tried to make certain that incompetents were not licensed to practice under its aegis. All three boards seemed to strive for objectivity. In 1894 the allopathic examiners failed 32.7 per cent, the homeopaths rejected 22 per cent, and the eclectics refused to pass a shocking 57.1 per cent of the candidates.[15]

The formation of separate boards, however, did not indicate that the orthodox profession was willing to accept homeopathy. Rather, it meant that the need for protection outweighed the differences between the sects. Allopathic intolerance did not disappear so easily. For an example, one need only look at the case of the Mount Vernon Hospital in Westchester, New York. The board of managers threatened to resign in 1893 rather than allow the appointment of homeopaths to the house staff. According to a humorous account in *Harper's Weekly*, the homeopaths "want a hack" at the patients. The editor noted that "there is only one thing that it is harder to get out of a hospital than an allopathic doctor, and that of course is his patient." Continuing in this vein, he conceded that many in the profession "cure now in a good many times wherein their predecessors usually killed," but they "now cost a great deal more." The article concluded by predicting that in the future "the homeopath and allopath will lie down together" to be treated by the Christian Scientist.[16]

The year after the trouble in Westchester, however, the recently established Association of American Medical Colleges officially recognized that the homeopathic schools were just as efficient in teaching the essentials of medicine as their orthodox counterparts. That body passed a by-law which provided that homeopathic graduates could be admitted to advanced standing, with every credit being accepted but those in strictly homeopathic subjects.[17]

In 1895 the past president of the Philadelphia County Medical Society, Dr. John B. Roberts, published a book entitled *Modern Medicine and Homeopathy*. This volume, according to the *New England Medical Gazette*, must have made the rabid allopaths of the past "restless in their graves."

[14] *New York Medical Journal* 52 (July 12, 1890): 46. For Pennsylvania's similar compromise, see *Hahnemannian Monthly* 28 (March 1893): 198–200; and (July 1893): 488–89.

[15] *New York Medical Journal* 41 (February 16, 1895): 212–13.

[16] "Differences between Doctors," *Harper's Weekly Magazine* 37 (November 11, 1893): 1086.

[17] *Bulletin of the American Academy of Medicine* 1 (August 1894): 532.

Roberts asserted that there was so little difference between the homeopathic and allopathic medicine that he regularly consulted with homeopaths. He concluded by noting that any physician could join the A.M.A., as long as he did not practice "exclusively according to the homeopathic law of similars."[18]

The next year, Roberts wrote an article critical of the orthodox attitude toward homeopathy. He declared that if homeopaths were allowed to rejoin the profession without being forced "down on their knees and confessing that they have been sinners," they would become "regular" in every sense of the term. The Philadelphia physician rhetorically asked why irregulars continued to preach homeopathy, yet did not seem to practice what they preached. He accounted for their actions by explaining that it was a form of self-defense.[19] That same year, an article in the *Journal of the American Medical Association* demonstrated why the homeopaths were always on the defensive. It asserted that Hahnemann was totally insane, and having abandoned his idiocy, the homeopaths now practiced "real medicine."[20] The insistence that homeopathy had descended from an "insane" theorist was hardly calculated to build bridges between the sects. Similarly, the assertion that homeopathy was merely an "expired trade-mark" angered the moderates who believed that homeopathy was a worth while addition to medical knowledge.

In a series on homeopathy, Dr. William E. Quine, a midwestern physician, added fuel to the fire. He suggested that a "real scientist" could not repudiate the ideas of a sect, yet claim to be a member of that sect. Since homeopaths had renounced the Hahnemannian tenets, Quine was convinced that homeopathy was nothing but a fraud. "There is nothing for them to unite upon," he said, "but the name 'Homeopath.'"[21] Such comments published in leading allopathic journals only served to alienate the most liberal irregulars, while demonstrating to the more intransigent ones that it was impossible to ally with the "bigoted" allopaths.[22]

In spite of the continuing enmity, a few orthodox medical societies

---

[18] John B. Roberts, *Modern Medicine and Homeopathy* (Philadelphia, 1895), pp. 10-11, 64. See also the review of that work in *New England Medical Gazette* 31 (January 1896): 35-38.

[19] John B. Roberts, "The Present Attitude of Physicians and Modern Medicine towards Homeopathy," *Journal of the A.M.A.* 26 (February 15, 1896): 299-307.

[20] W. W. Parker, "Was Hahnemann Insane?" *Journal of the A.M.A.* 26 (January 4, 1896): 7-9.

[21] William E. Quine, "The Medical Profession," *Journal of the A.M.A.* 32 (April 29, 1899): 980.

[22] See for instance the reaction to a similar article, in *Hahnemannian Monthly* 33 (April 1898): 258-62.

began to pave the way for the eventual merger of the two groups. In 1888 the councillors of the Massachusetts Medical Society went even further than their New York colleagues had during the new-code controversy. They voted to allow graduates of homeopathic colleges to be examined for admittance to fellowship. To join the society, however, the candidate had to repudiate homeopathy, publicly renounce its every tenet, and practically assert that he had been living in sin.[23] This was a high price to pay for entrance into orthodox society, yet it did represent an advance. The society was in effect admitting that homeopathic colleges were not at all inferior to allopathic ones. Homeopathic degrees were henceforth equal to orthodox diplomas as evidence of professional attainment.

Despite the olive branch offered by the Massachusetts allopaths, most homeopaths were in no rush to abandon their heritage. Yet, the willingness of a few to recant led to increased bitterness and strife within the homeopathic ranks. The first evidence of division came with the demand for changes in the staff of the Ward's Island Hospital in New York City. In 1875 the commissioners of charities and correction had assigned that hospital to the county homeopathic society, which had petitioned for the "right" to treat the insane in a public institution.[24] In 1889, after fourteen years of operation, the Society insisted that the commissioners replace the entire medical board with physicians more committed to homeopathy.

The problem centered around Egbert Guernsey, an outspoken individual who seemed to be in the midst of every homeopathic dispute. As president of the Ward's Island staff, he had alienated the conservative faction by asserting that the law of similars was "important," but "not of universal application." He then outraged all but a handful of his colleagues when he advocated the elimination of the name "homeopathy" because of its bad connotation. In its place, he suggested that homeopaths call themselves the "new school," a name which implied scientific advances.

On January 2, 1890, the hospital board responded to the demand for change by passing a resolution declaring that it would be "a dangerous proceeding to permit a Medical Society, dominated as it often is by intensely personal feeling, to control the medical board of a public hospital." In addition, the board asserted that although the requirement for appointment

[23] Massachusetts Medical Society, *A Catalogue of Its Officers, Fellows, and Licentiates, 1781–1893* (Boston, 1894), p. 29; *New England Medical Gazette* 23 (March 1888): 101–3.
[24] *New York Times*, September 6, 1875, p. 8, col. 2; *New York Daily Tribune*, September 11, 1875, p. 12, col. 1.

to the staff should be a belief in *similia*, every physician should be able to "make use of any established principle in medical science."[25] When the commissioners refused to take action, Dr. J. M. Schley, an officer of the county society, declared that Guernsey would be taught a valuable lesson, as "soon as legal ground for his expulsion could be found."[26]

On February 5 Guernsey found himself on trial on several counts at a special meeting of the Society. First, the prosecution declared that he had told a *New York Sun* reporter that the Society was "unworthy and dishonest." Guernsey insisted that he was correct when he made this assessment of the Society's role in the Ward's Island dispute. Next, he was accused of telling a representative of the *Evening Post* that the actions of the Society were based "not upon truth but upon misrepresentation and falsehood." He declared that he had been misquoted. The third charge was that he had published a devastating attack upon Dr. T. F. Allen, who had introduced a resolution to remove Guernsey's *Medical Times* from the list of publications approved by the American Institute of Homeopathy. Finally, he was charged with having asserted that all homeopaths were "dishonest and deceitful." At the trial, he denied that the Society had any power to discipline him, calling it a "Star Chamber" and a medical "inquisition."[27] As might be expected, Guernsey was found guilty and expelled from the Society.

East Coast homeopaths were not the only ones facing internal dissension. Officers of the Hahnemann Medical College of San Francisco suddenly repudiated homeopathy and announced that they intended to affiliate with an orthodox college. The editor of the *Hahnemannian Monthly* asserted that homeopathy was better off without such incompetents, who "will leave behind them a purified atmosphere and a host of earnest workers."[28]

In 1893 a similar situation occurred in the midwest. Dr. H. L. Obetz, dean of the homeopathic division of the University of Michigan, asserted that the homeopathic school should be merged with the allopathic one. Over the years, a virtually independent homeopathic college had emerged side by side with the orthodox one. Since homeopathic and allopathic practices were growing increasingly alike, it was a waste of money for the taxpayers to be supporting two identical schools with separate professors

[25] *New York Medical Times* 17 (February 1890): 343–44; *New York Times*, January 7, 1890, p. 8, col. 4.

[26] *New York Times*, December 13, 1889, p. 3, cols. 4–5; December 14, 1889, p. 1, cols. 5–6.

[27] *New York Medical Times* 17 (March 1890): 373–74.

[28] *Hahnemannian Monthly* 29 (May 1894): 294–95.

and classes in Ann Arbor. Regardless of the logic behind his proposal, "Judas" Obetz was universally condemned by his fellow homeopaths. In fact, the American Institute of Homeopathy passed a resolution insisting that he be relieved of his duties for being so unfaithful to the cause.[29]

After a great deal of discussion, the regents decided that the homeopathic faculty, by demanding that the dean be fired from his position, was attempting to dictate policy. In consequence, the resignation of the entire homeopathic staff was requested. The college was continued on its old basis, with a completely different homeopathic faculty.[30]

With the division of the orthodox profession into liberal and conservative wings over the consultation issue, it was natural for the homeopathic demands of the past to be reconsidered. When so many prominent allopaths were willing to accept homeopaths as legitimate practitioners, it seemed ridiculous to continue to deny their "rights" to hospital facilities and to appointment in the military. Allopaths who earlier had refused to let homeopathic treatment invade their wards slowly came to realize that, like it or not, homeopathy was legal, somewhat popular, and apparently a permanent feature of American medicine.

Chicago provided an excellent example of the changing public attitude wrought by the evolution of practice and the consultation dispute. As noted in chapter five, during the 1850's the city fathers had allowed the new city hospital to stand empty rather than to turn it over to the homeopaths. On November 28, 1881, however, after the alterations in practice had become widely known, a committee of the board of county commissioners recommended that homeopathy be introduced into the Cook County Hospital. Following a short debate, it was decided to let the homeopaths control one fifth of the wards, with the patients being assigned at random.[31]

On this occasion, the allopaths did not threaten to resign rather than associate with irregular practitioners. Instead, they claimed that every citizen should have the right to select his own type of treatment. When the homeopaths expressed no objection, the committee on hospitals unanimously revised the original plan. By May, however, the committee was

[29] Burke A. Hinsdale, *History of the University of Michigan* (Ann Arbor, 1906), p. 110; J. C. Nottingham to J. B. Angell, Bay City, Michigan, April 15, 1893, MS in Angell Papers, Michigan Historical Collection.

[30] Regents, *Proceedings, 1891–1896*, pp. 379–80, 513–14.

[31] *Chicago Herald*, November 29, 1881, p. 1, col. 7; *Daily Inter Ocean* (Chicago), November 29, 1881, p. 8, col. 3. See also the report of the episode in Chicago Medical Society, *History of Medicine and Surgery...of Chicago* (Chicago, 1922), pp. 215–26, 267.

informed that the average patient "does not actually know the difference between homeopathic and regular school treatment." To solve that problem, the homeopaths were given every fourth male surgical and female gynecological patient, along with every fifth medical case,[32] and were quite at home sharing the facilities at Cook County Hospital.

One result of this arrangement was that it provided a comparison between regular and homeopathic treatment for a period of time. For the year ending August 31, 1884, for instance, the allopaths treated 4,692 cases, losing 8.6 per cent. Over the same period, the homeopaths handled 1,242 patients, with 8.2 per cent failing to recover. For a sixteen month period in 1886 and 1887, the allopaths reported a mortality of 7.2 per cent, while the homeopathic division lost 8.7 per cent. When separated into their medical and surgical components, the evidence indicates that the homeopaths did better surgically. That may be explained by the fact that they used the knife only in obviously surgical cases. On the other hand, orthodox physicians did decidedly better medically, which may be explained by the fact that in treating medically, the homeopaths lost a number of patients who might have profited from surgery.[33]

Although the cases were chosen at random, the resulting statistics are in no sense definitive. First, there is no way of determining the degree of the homeopathic treatment. Was it pure homeopathy, or did it include many aspects of the allopathic practice? A more accurate clinical evaluation could have been made on the basis of a number of similar cases, with half treated by each system, using double-blind techniques. Unfortunately, few physicians of either school would have allowed "improper" treatment of their patients, so an evaluation of this type was never attempted.

Boston provided another example of the changing attitude toward homeopathy that accompanied the evolution of medical practice. At a time when only a few citizens were aware of the narrowing gap between homeopathic and allopathic practices, the faculty of the Boston University School of Medicine petitioned for permission to use the facilities of the Boston City Hospital for clinical instruction. Since the students at the Harvard Medical School had already been granted this right, the hospital trustees could scarcely reject the homeopathic request.[34]

[32] Cook County Board of Commissioners, *Proceedings, 1881–1882* (Chicago, n.d.), pp. 28–29, 222–23.
[33] Cook County Hospital, *Annual Report, 1884* (Chicago, 1885), pp. 24–28; *Annual Report, 1887* (Chicago, 1888), pp. 8, 15.
[34] *New England Medical Gazette* 21 (November 1886): 514.

The allopathic medical board, however, was vehement in its opposition to any homeopathic incursion, and at one point the entire staff threatened to resign if irregulars were allowed in the hospital. The homeopaths could not believe that the orthodox profession would be so foolish as to hand over the hospital by a mass resignation. One homeopath exclaimed: "We do not give them the credit for being . . . such asses. What a glorious opportunity it would be for us!"[35] The trustees finally decided that the petition could not be granted and homeopathy continued to be excluded from the wards of Boston City Hospital.

In 1885 the Boston University faculty renewed its demands, but by this time the new-code controversy had demonstrated that conditions had changed. Interestingly, on July 21 not one person appeared to condemn the proposal. Apparently, the trustees could not believe that the orthodox practitioners had intended to remain silent, so a second hearing was scheduled on February 19, 1886, at which the only opposition came from the members of the staff. After a number of months had elapsed, the trustees adopted a report which declared that "as the hospital is a city institution," they "cannot invite students of one school, and debar those of another." This meant that homeopathic students would be able to visit the wards for clinical observation, as long as they did not interfere with treatment. Since a number of the students were women, the trustees agreed for the first time to allow females to visit both the wards and the surgical amphitheater.[36]

Just as the attitude of the hospital boards had changed from one of complete opposition to the introduction of homeopathy to a policy of silent toleration, the government medical service experienced a similar transformation. It will be recalled that during the American Civil War, homeopaths unsuccessfully had fought for appointment to the Union medical corps.[37] In 1882 they were still demanding the "right" to take the entrance examinations. Dr. J. C. Morgan, chairman of the Bureau of Medical Legislation of the American Institute of Homeopathy, wrote to ask Congressman Charles O'Neill if sectarians still faced discrimination in the federal service. His letter was forwarded to the secretaries of the army and navy. The secretary of the navy soon replied that no "discrimination is made in favor of or against any school." Appointment to the naval medical corps was by competitive examination based upon knowledge and ability.

In the case of the army, the situation was more familiar. Surgeon-General

---

[35] Ibid. 15 (April 1880): 97–99.
[36] Ibid. 21 (November 1886): 514–18.
[37] See chapter five.

Barnes reported that the term "regular," as applied to medical schools, referred to the quality of education rather than to legal standing. The knowledge expected of a surgical or medical officer, he explained, could not be acquired at an "irregular" school. He declared that, as a matter of policy, "it is not considered desirable to introduce in the army the practice of homeopathy . . . or any other *sectarian and exclusive* system of medicine." Although the homeopaths sought to change this decision, they were unsuccessful.[38]

By the time of the Spanish-American War, however, the attitude of the army had changed considerably. Angered when they learned that homeopaths were still being refused examination by state medical boards, a number of Philadelphia homeopaths appealed to the United States Congress and to President William McKinley. The latter ordered that all physicians who applied for commissions should be examined, and those who could pass should be enrolled into the military. Surgeon-General Von Ripen reportedly was pleased at the addition of homeopathic practitioners. He was primarily interested in reducing expenses, and homeopathic medication was known to be inexpensive.[39]

Despite the many gains made by the homeopathic practitioners, complete toleration of their school was still in the future. Before any further progress could be made, the medical profession had to revise its code of ethics. During the first few years of the new century, the regular physicians sought to eliminate the differences in their own ranks. The reorganization of the A.M.A. had to be completed as the first step in this process. Professional unity could only be accomplished by coming to terms with the consultation question, the issue which had originally brought the New York liberals into conflict with the national fraternity.

In 1900 the A.M.A. appointed a committee to study its changing organizational needs. Under the existing system, the "general meeting," which possessed legislative functions, seated virtually every physician who happened to attend the annual convention. This meant that physicians in nearby states maintained the preponderance of power. The annual conventions, then, were never truly representative. The committee on reorganization recommended that representation be set at one delegate for every five hundred members, and that the basic unit be the county medical society. A new creation, the "house of delegates," would more equitably represent the

---

[38] *New England Medical Gazette* 17 (December 1882): 353–56.
[39] *Journal of the A.M.A.* 30 (June 11, 1898): 1430; *North American Journal of Homeopathy* 3d ser., 13 (June 1898): 380–82; (August 1898): 519–20.

state and local constituents. The adoption of this report insured that the A.M.A. conventions of the future would be national in scope and that the association could speak for the orthodox profession.[40]

At the first meeting after reorganization, at Saratoga Springs, New York, Dr. E. Eliot Harris reported that his committee of the New York State Medical Association had critically analyzed and revised the code of ethics, subject, of course, to the approval of the house of delegates. The president of the A.M.A., New York's Dr. John A. Wyeth, appointed an eminent five-man committee to investigate the "principles of ethics" suggested by the state association. The committee included several of the leading and most familiar names in American medicine, men such as the founder of the Johns Hopkins Medical College, Dr. William H. Welch, and Nicholas Senn, Chicago's master of abdominal surgery.[41] The fact that individuals of this caliber were named to the committee indicates the high priority given to bringing the New York profession back into the fold.

Meanwhile, the two New York state societies had appointed their own committees to discuss a possible merger. On December 19, 1902, they met with Dr. Frank Billings, the new president of the A.M.A., who told them that while the old code was still in force, it was no longer binding upon the state societies.[42] When the A.M.A. met at New Orleans in 1903, it replaced the old code with an "advisory document," largely written by Welch. Whereas the old code was law, the advisory document was merely a statement of principles. On the vital consultation issue, it declared: "The broadest dictates of humanity should be obeyed by physicians whenever and wherever their services are needed to meet the emergencies of disease or accident." This statement brought the A.M.A. fully in line with the Medical Society of the State of New York, and it paved the way for reunification of the orthodox medical profession, an event which took place during the next two years.[43]

In addition to tempering the A.M.A. stand upon the consultation issue, the advisory document authorized the local societies to admit all legally recognized practitioners. The net effect of this clause was to admit home-

[40] Morris Fishbein, *A History of the A.M.A.* (Philadelphia and London, 1947), pp. 204–13. *New York Daily Tribune*, November 29, 1901, p. 7, cols. 3–4.

[41] Fishbein, *History of the A.M.A.*, p. 222; *Journal of the A.M.A.* 38 (June 21, 1902): 1649–52.

[42] *New York Medical Journal* 77 (February 7, 1903): 259–64.

[43] Fishbein, *History of the A.M.A.*, pp. 227–28, 238; *New York Times*, May 17, 1903, p. 30, cols. 1–3; *New York Medical Journal* 78 (October 17, 1903): 756.

opaths.[44] The *Journal of the American Medical Association* was soon asked by several societies whether or not they could or should admit irregulars. The editor stated in response that according to both the reorganization plan and the code of ethics, any registered physician of good moral character, who does not "support or practice, or claim to practice, any exclusive system of medicine" shall be eligible for membership. The fact that he may have graduated from an irregular college no longer could prevent his enrollment. The editor went on to recommend that homeopaths be accepted. "It may be better, in some instances, to admit them than to reject one whose status is not perfectly clear, because the very admission, through its fellowship with men of high professional ideals, may prove the turning point of a career begun in error and continued for the lack of opportunity to retrace false steps taken in ignorance and innocence."[45]

By 1903 the orthodox profession was united under the A.M.A., and homeopaths wishing to take advantage of the scientific and professional benefits of that society, and willing to recant, could join. The allopaths had drastically altered their stand, although it is clear that some apparently advocated the admission of homeopaths simply in order to destroy their system by submerging it in orthodoxy. Despite the increasing toleration of homeopathy, the orthodox profession continued to consider the homeopath as a "deceived" man whose career was "begun in error," and who was unable to "retrace false steps taken in ignorance and innocence."

[44] *Hahnemannian Monthly* 38 (July 1903): 538–39.
[45] *Journal of the A.M.A.* 43 (October 15, 1904): 1158–59.

XI

PROGRESSIVISM AND THE DECLINE OF HOMEOPATHY

Now that the A.M.A. had finally decided to admit irregular practitioners, the homeopathic profession was faced with a new set of problems. One possible result of the merger with orthodoxy was the loss of homeopathic identity, and homeopaths could scarcely be expected to endorse a plan which might destroy the reasons for their own existence. In addition to the difficulties implicit in merger, the reorganization of the A.M.A. paved the way for a full-scale drive to improve medical education, a movement which proved detrimental to homeopathy by demonstrating that the irregular colleges were inferior, incapable of preparing students for the medical licensing examinations.

Dr. William Osler, long the leading physician in America, and one of the more respected allopaths, asserted in 1905 that homeopathic and allopathic practices were so similar that the orthodox profession should not insist that there was any distinction between regular and irregular colleges. "A difference in drugs should no longer separate men with the same hope. The original quarrel is ours," he admitted, "but the homeopaths should not allow themselves to be separated by a shibboleth that is inconsistent with their practice today." [1]

Osler's plea was for his colleagues to open the door of orthodoxy to the irregulars. Unfortunately, few homeopaths were anxious to accept any overture from the traditionally intolerant allopaths. The editor of the *Hahnemannian Monthly* noted that Osler was fair-minded, but until others manifested a similar spirit "attempts at unity between the two schools will

[1] *New York Times*, April 28, 1905, p. 6, col. 1.

be fruitless." Until homeopathic therapeutics were accepted, "it is the duty of our school," he said, "to preserve and develop the principles of homeopathy."[2]

In 1906 Dr. Frederick C. Shattuck joined Osler in extending the hand of friendship to his unorthodox colleagues. At a meeting of the Boston Homeopathic Society, the professor of clinical medicine at Harvard Medical School read a paper in which he declared that the orthodox physicians should seek "to do no harm in treatment." During the development of therapeutic nihilism in the United States, toward the end of the nineteenth century, many advocates of mild medication recognized, along with Shattuck, that the effects of their practices were similar to those of the highly diluted homeopathic doses. Shattuck told his homeopathic audience that he hoped that a state society encompassing the two sects could be established in Massachusetts. In reporting Shattuck's suggestions, the *Hahnemannian Monthly* noted: "Our friends, the enemy" are offering the olive branch. Despite the scientific attitude of the Bostonian, the editor predicted that all attempts at merger would fail because of the decades of mutual distrust.[3]

In 1906 another allopath, Dr. Richard C. Cabot, went quite a bit further than had Osler or Shattuck. Cabot admitted, as did Osler before him, that his school had traditionally been "in the wrong." Allopathy, he said, had "receded from more false positions" than had the followers of Hahnemann. The waning popularity of blood-letting was evidence of the errors of the allopathic past. Cabot declared that orthodox practitioners should have never refused to consult with homeopaths, but, he said, "we have seen and admitted our wrong." In addition, he asserted that the allopaths were foolish to call themselves "regular," an action which had implied that nonconformists were "irregular" and thus misguided. Finally, Cabot admitted that the orthodox profession should have been willing to experiment with homeopathic remedies. The question should have been "do they work," he exclaimed, rather than "are they logical."[4]

Beginning in 1908 several homeopaths tried to remedy the situation by convincing the American Medical Association to investigate the law of similars. Brooklyn's Dr. H. D. Schenck worked for two years in an attempt to persuade the A.M.A. to appoint a committee to work with a similar one of the American Institute of Homeopathy. Dr. J. N. McCormack, the

---

[2] *Hahnemannian Monthly* 40 (October 1905): 773–75.
[3] Ibid. 41 (May 1906): 374–78.
[4] *New England Medical Gazette* 41 (December 1906): 587–95.

Kentuckian who was the driving force behind the 1903 reorganization of the A.M.A., reportedly told his colleagues: "We must admit that we have never fought the homeopath on matters of principles; we fought him because he came into the community and got the business."[5] Science and medicine, then, demanded an experiment with the law of similars.

In 1913 the homeopaths managed to convince Dr. Abraham Jacobi, at that time the president of the A.M.A., to use his influence to encourage the national fraternity to co-operate in an investigation of homeopathic therapeutics. Under the plan accepted by both associations the testing was to be done under the auspices of the Rockefeller Institute of New York or the McCormack Institute of Chicago. The A.I.H. declared in an open letter that if the laws of homeopathy "be proven true, humanity will be benefited by the enlarged and improved armamentarium of all physicians; if it be disproven, the last obstacle to medical union will have been removed."[6] The test was never to be completed, however; Dr. Alexander R. Craig, secretary of the A.M.A., was soon to inform the homeopaths that the two institutes had refused to participate in the experiment. Craig asked the A.I.H. to suggest other acceptable laboratories. At that point, the homeopaths decided to drop the matter; for some reason, Craig's letter was interpreted as demonstrating little enthusiasm for the project.[7]

Despite the well-meaning attempts to unite the sects in a common brotherhood, as seen in the remarks of Cabot, Shattuck, and Osler, and the movement to investigate the scientific merits of homeopathy, many allopaths continued to exhibit intolerance and bigotry. This intransigence cast doubt upon the good intentions of the liberal members of the orthodox school. One example was publicized by the editor of the *Hahnemannian Monthly*. He discovered that when the *Journal of the American Medical Association* printed an obituary of a converted homeopath, it invariably neglected to name his alma mater. The *Monthly* editor exclaimed that the comment of Reverend Robert Hall toward a member of his congregation was quite relevant to the editor of the *Journal*. "He has a soul so small that it could be put in a nut-shell; and moreover, if there was a maggot hole in the shell, it would drop out."[8]

The editor of the *Journal of the American Medical Association*, Dr.

[5] Quoted in *Journal of the American Institute of Homeopathy* 4 (May 1912): 1359–60.

[6] Ibid. 6 (October 1913): 337–41.

[7] Ibid. 8 (September 1915): 327–28.

[8] *Hahnemannian Monthly* 40 (November 1905): 856–57.

George H. Simmons, was a graduate of the Hahnemann Medical College of Chicago. He had practiced homeopathy for ten years and then converted to orthodoxy.[9] To the more conservative Hahnemannians, Simmons was a traitor of the first order; his treatment of homeopathy as editor of the leading allopathic magazine reinforced their opinion. Simmons published a number of articles uncomplimentary to his former practice. Since this was hardly in line with the drive to unite the profession under the banner of orthodoxy, it demonstrated to many homeopaths that the merger proposal was a ruse intended to destroy homeopathy. In February of 1913, Simmons accepted an article in which the author undiplomatically declared: "Of all the medical systems of present or past times, there is none which in my opinion has a scantier basis of fact or reason, a poorer excuse for existence, or a more fantastic set of principles and methods, than Homeopathy."[10]

In reaction to the denunciatory articles, America's homeopaths closed ranks. In 1904 Dr. Eldridge C. Price told the Maryland State Homeopathic Medical Society that since the homeopaths were popular, self-sufficient, and scientifically correct, they could gain nothing from affiliating with orthodox practitioners. Well aware of the answer, Price asked whether irregulars who joined the A.M.A. would be able to discuss homeopathic therapeutics at allopathic conventions.[11] The editor of the *Maryland Medical Journal* noted quite correctly that the homeopaths were faced with the possibility of voting themselves out of existence in order to maintain or spread the truths of their sect. To the homeopath, it would be foolish "to risk the disintegration of his party for the sake of propagating his faith." "It would be a great triumph" if homeopaths were able to add their knowledge to the orthodox, "but very poor politics."[12] In response to the comments of Price and the editorial of the Maryland journal, the *Hahnemannian Monthly* asserted that homeopathy was slowly being accepted as orthodox practice, so there was no need to affiliate with allopaths. Indeed, merger would only serve to "water-down the truth."[13]

Dr. De Witt Wilcox, of Buffalo and later Boston, in his 1906 presidential address before the Homeopathic Medical Society of the State of New York, also asserted that the only way to effect a viable union between the sects would be for the allopaths to examine and publicly report on the

---

[9] Ibid. 41 (January 1906): 59; see also the Simmons' biography in Morris Fishbein, *A History of the A.M.A.* (Philadelphia and London, 1941), pp. 350–57.
[10] *Journal of the A.M.A.* 60 (February 1, 1913): 331–37.
[11] *Maryland Medical Journal* 47 (July 1904): 255–62.
[12] Ibid., pp. 276–77.
[13] *Hahnemannian Monthly* 39 (August 1904): 611–15.

claims of homeopathy. "If we become a part of the dominant school, then our *principles* must become a part of them." [14]

In 1907 the Philadelphia County Medical Society adopted a resolution opening its doors to any physician who agreed "not to accept any sectarian designation or base his practice upon any exclusive dogma or system." Homeopaths were so suspicious of their allopathic colleagues that the editor of the *Hahnemannian Monthly* tried to determine the motivation behind this unexpected action. It was unlikely, he said, that it indicated repentence for past intolerance, especially since Philadelphia had always been known as a center of medical bigotry. The editor then suggested that since the legalization of consultations would add to the income of specialists, economics was one reason for this action. He also suggested that the olive branch might have been offered as a "pretence of liberality which will enable the dominant school to drive the homeopathic profession out of existence as an organized body." Finally, he predicted that the proposed merger would be the forerunner of a legislative fight to enact a one-board licensure bill.[15]

Reacting defensively, many homeopaths demanded a return to the practice of Hahnemann, meaning the acceptance of pure homeopathy. A Maryland homeopath, for instance, complained that a major problem was that so many of his colleagues were homeopaths in name only. The colleges, he said, taught totally inadequate courses in therapeutics and *materia medica*.[16] The 1910 convention of the A.I.H. debated a proposal which demanded that in order to combat the attempt of the A.M.A. to destroy homeopathy, all members who enrolled in allopathic societies should be expelled from homeopathic ones.[17] Since this action might eventually depopulate the national homeopathic institute, the resolution was tabled.

Although the proposal was defeated, homeopaths who wanted to ally with the orthodox profession were condemned as "heretics" and "traitors." One such physician was Dr. Charles E. Kahlke, the president of the Illinois Homeopathic Medical Association and the dean of Chicago's Hahnemann Medical College. He was so "unpatriotic" that he censured his fellow homeopaths for failing to keep abreast of the scientific advances of the day, and he insisted that there would eventually be a mutually beneficial merger. Kahlke was denounced by the conservative homeopathic faction, who

[14] *New England Medical Gazette* 41 (May 1906): 248–49.
[15] *Hahnemannian Monthly* 41 (November 1907): 855–61.
[16] W. L. Morgan, "The Disintegration of the Homeopathic Profession," *Homeopathic Recorder* 24 (August 15, 1909): 339–43.
[17] *Journal of the American Institute of Homeopathy* 3 (November 1910): 257.

initiated a drive to establish a society to carry out the principles of "true homeopathy."[18]

Between 1900 and 1906 the members of the A.M.A. came to believe that society had to be protected from the newer medical sects—the osteopaths, chiropractors, and Christian Scientists. The three-board medical examining system was a bad precedent; newer groups were demanding the right to regulate their own practices through the establishment of additional boards. Acceding to this demand would have destroyed the national licensure system, since with each sect setting its own standards, the public would no longer be protected from incompetent physicians. The allopaths were convinced that one of the many boards would certainly license unqualified applicants, and at this time a great many of the osteopaths, chiropractors, and Christian Scientists had received little or no medical training.

In 1903 New Jersey's homeopaths and allopaths united to oppose an osteopathic licensure bill. The state, however, already had a unified board. In those states with two or three separate boards, the demand for additional examining boards threatened the destruction of the entire system. The only alternative was to establish combined allopathic-homeopathic-eclectic boards which would pass upon the applications of Christian Scientists, osteopaths, and chiropractors. This would insure that every physician was well-versed in anatomy, physiology, and other medical subjects.[19]

In 1907 the *New York Times* declared that "One Board is Enough." In an editorial it warned that if the older sects did not consolidate the three boards, the osteopaths and Christian Scientists would soon have their own examiners. If the allopaths and homeopaths were unwilling to surrender their autonomy, the *Times* predicted that "they will see the whole state licensing system reduced to a farce and the public's protection from quacks destroyed."[20]

In the case of New York, the agitation for unified boards led to a bitter fight between the more respectable sects and the newcomers to medical science, especially the more numerous and relatively better educated osteopaths. Finally, in 1907 the legislature passed a bill which provided for a nine-man board to examine all applicants on the entire spectrum of medical science. Therapeutics and *materia medica*, however, would not be tested, as

---

[18] *Chicago Record-Herald*, May 12, 1911, p. 9, col. 2; June 7, 1911, p. 3, col. 4.
[19] *Hahnemannian Monthly* 41 (March 1907): 217-21; David L. Cowen, *Medicine and Health in New Jersey: A History* (Princeton, 1964), pp. 74, 129.
[20] *New York Times*, February 26, 1907, p. 10, col. 4.

homeopaths and eclectics refused to be tested in their own specialty by a board with an allopathic majority. Proficiency in those subjects would be certified by the individual medical colleges. In order to further eliminate any possibility of favoritism, examination was to be by number rather than by name. In addition, only graduates of colleges having four-year courses of study could present themselves for examination. Moreover, those schools had to abide by guidelines governing premedical education.[21]

The bill was intended to insure that every New York physician had an adequate background, had graduated from a recognized college, and was competent in the basic medical fields. Interestingly, in the process it legalized the practice of osteopathy and other smaller sects. Any graduate of a recognized school with a four-year course who was capable of passing the examination would have to be licensed. The bill, an excellent one, provided the basis for complete protection from quacks and charlatans.

In 1910 relations between the sects were shaken by the proposed Owen Bill, which would have established a federal department of health with broad discretionary powers. The A.M.A. joined a number of public health organizations in advocating immediate passage of the bill. Since the A.M.A. had taken so strong a stand, many homeopaths became convinced that there must have been something evil about the bill. They thought that it was another attempt of the allopaths to destroy competition. According to this line of thought, the department of health might prohibit physicians from dispensing drugs. That would have destroyed homeopathy, since homeopaths had always carried and administered their own medications. The drive to establish a federal health department was seen by many irregulars as the next logical step in the A.M.A. attempt to control medical licensure.[22]

The unorthodox practitioners were not the only Americans who opposed public health laws. The National League for Medical Freedom suddenly appeared on the scene and soon became the spokesman for those who sought to prevent the passage of progressive legislation. The League was composed of patent medicine manufacturers, Christian Scientists, osteopaths, and a few homeopaths.[23] An exposé in *Collier's Weekly* demonstrated the diverse interests of those operating under the cloak of "Medical

[21] *Medical Record* 71 (May 18, 1907): 820; *Hahnemannian Monthly* 41 (June 1907): 463–66; (September 1907): 683–94; *Journal of the A.M.A.* 49 (November 30, 1907): 1867.
[22] *North American Journal of Homeopathy*, 3d ser., 25 (November 1910): 741–43.
[23] *Chicago Record-Herald*, November 22, 1911, p. 14, col. 4.

Freedom." B. O. Flower, one of the founders of the League, was the vociferous editor of the *Arena*, a muckraking magazine which fought for liberal and radical ideas, but which opposed public health legislation. He also had been president of the R. C. Flower Medicine Company from 1885 to 1899; so he had a direct financial interest in the war against the restrictive drug laws.

The next significant figure in the National League for Medical Freedom was the second vice president, an interesting character named C. W. Miller. Formerly a member of the Iowa legislature, he had become famous for his condemnation of public health laws. In 1909, although present in the assembly chamber, Miller was reported as either "absent or not voting" when a bill to strengthen the pure food laws passed by a vote of 70 to 0. Later, he voted against a more stringent measure. According to *Collier's*, Miller was made a director of the League as a result of his "record" in the legislature.[24]

Another founder of the League was Mrs. Diana Belais, who also served as president of an anti-vivisectionist society. *Collier's* described her as a "well-meaning, ignorant, reckless, and muddle-headed agitator." Dr. C. S. Carr, the editor of the obscure *Columbus Medical Journal*, was on the League's advisory board. Carr's magazine was hardly the epitome of scientific medicine. The May 1909 issue, for instance, included a cover photograph of Carr, along with the captions: "All drugs are poison. All druggists are poisoners." Other leaders in the fight against public health legislation were the patent medicine interests, who apparently were financing the League. In order to enlist additional workers, the League opposed medical licensure and so was able to attract a number of irregular practitioners.[25]

The advocates of "Medical Freedom" were quick to condemn every "misuse" of governmental authority in the field of public health. For instance, when "Typhoid Mary" Malon was hospitalized by the New York authorities, an eclectic physician who urged his colleagues to join the League complained that a "PERFECTLY HEALTHY girl is condemned as a 'germ factory' and deprived of her right of liberty and the pursuit of happiness."[26]

By the autumn of 1910, however, blind opposition to the Owen bill gave way to a more reasonable homeopathic attitude. Many homeopaths realized

---

[24] *Collier's Weekly Magazine* 47 (June 19, 1911): 9–10.
[25] Ibid.
[26] *California Eclectic Medical Journal* 3 (December 1910): 323.

that the government had an obligation to improve and protect the health of the nation.[27] The *North American Journal of Homeopathy* repudiated those homeopathic physicians whose "A-M-A-phobia is acute enough to have led them into flirting with the so-called League for Medical Freedom." The editor insisted that the League was contrary to the ideals of the medical profession. One homeopath who had attended a meeting of the Denver branch of the League reported that he heard a "loud-mouthed, blatant demagogue of a blatherskite practically pronounce the medical profession a band of murderers." Three-quarters of the deaths in Denver were "attributed to the medical profession of that city."[28]

The delegates to the 1910 convention of the American Institute of Homeopathy discussed the Owen bill. Dr. Lewis P. Crutcher, of Kansas City, considered it an attempt of the allopaths to eliminate competition. "It means you must either join the A.M.A., or get off the M.A.P." Philadelphia's Dr. Thomas Carmichael declared that the proposed department of public health would destroy the free enterprise system. Dr. Joseph Hensley of Oklahoma City suggested that the homeopaths scream "trust" when the bill finally reached the floor of Congress. As every "moral" and "patriotic" American was opposed to monopolistic business practices, Hensley believed that the cry of "trust" would force the legislators to vote against the bill. Other homeopaths asserted that the A.M.A. was the largest and most irresponsible trust in the United States. In rebuttal, New York's Dr. Hills Cole, a member of the American Public Health Association, insisted that the Owen bill was intended to protect the nation's health and that it was not intended to destroy homeopathy. After all the debate, the A.I.H. passed a resolution in favor of "proper health legislation," and it established a committee to draft a more acceptable bill.[29]

During the search for an acceptable response, an "Uncle Remus" type of commentary appeared in several homeopathic and eclectic journals. Brer Fox, the allopath, was jealous of the popularity and success of Brer Rabbit, the irregular practitioner. In order to stunt the future growth of rabbits, Brer Fox refused to meet them in professional consultation. When he recognized that Brer Rabbit was strengthened by persecution, Brer Fox changed his tactics. He decided to control medical licensure by enacting legislation compelling every physician to pass an examination administered

[27] *North American Journal of Homeopathy*, 3d ser., 25 (July 1910): 478–80.
[28] Ibid. (December 1910): 811–14.
[29] *Journal of the American Institute of Homeopathy* 3 (November 1910): 249–56.

by a board "of Brer Fox's own choosing." That scheme could have worked perfectly, if only foxes were on the board, but "a generous and fair-minded public said: 'Rabbits have just as good rights in this briar patch as foxes, and if license boards exist, rabbits shall be represented upon them.'" Frustrated by the will of the people, Brer Fox decided to take a different tack. He declared: "What we need, Brer Rabbit, is a great Department of Public Health with a wise old Fox at the head of it who should have absolute authority to do anything he pleased in sanitary affairs," meaning, of course, passage of the Owen bill. Brer Hawkeye of the National League for Medical Freedom entered the scene at that point, declaring that the Owen bill was "just a coypigeon to fool the people while Brer Fox bags the game." [30]

Although the American Institute of Homeopathy hesitated to align itself with a potentially dangerous ally like the League for Medical Freedom, most homeopaths did agree with its position on licensure. The League actively tried to recruit homeopathic aid, but failed to enroll more than a few Hahnemannians. One who did become involved was Dr. John B. Garrison, an official of the A.I.H., who gave permission for the League to use his name on their circulars. A letter condemning the proposed national bureau of health, signed by Garrison and Royal Copeland, a homeopath later to become United States Senator from New York, was circulated to the homeopathic profession of that state. In a letter to the editor of the *North American Journal of Homeopathy*, Garrison admitted that he knew nothing about what the League represented, or where it got its funds. "I am not in sympathy with all its methods," he declared, "but I am glad of the help it is giving in the way of publicity." [31]

The influential Dr. De Witt Wilcox was bitterly opposed to any alliance with those who sought "to annul or belittle" all the great medical advances of the last several decades. The League advocated the abolition of the state and local boards of health, and it denied that quarantine of infectious diseases was necessary. Moreover, it condemned the medical program for school children as an unnecessary and unconstitutional restriction upon individual liberty. Wilcox even went so far as to assert that if homeopaths

---

[30] *California Eclectic Medical Journal* 4 (February 1911): 60–63; *North American Journal of Homeopathy*, 3d ser., 25 (December 1910): 814–18.

[31] *North American Journal of Homeopathy* 58 (November 1910): 746–48; (December 1910), 811–14. Unlike the American Institute of Homeopathy, The National Eclectic Medical Association voted to thank the League for its work in the cause of medical freedom. See *N.E.M.A. Quarterly* 3 (September 1911): 19 and 34.

were "so afraid that the dominant school will legislate us out of business that we must call to our aid the medical quacks, the Christian scientists, the poison food squad, and all the other medical sore-heads . . . it is better that we die a respectable death and have a decent burial." [32]

The *Homeopathic Recorder* disagreed with the Wilcox analysis. Since the Owen bill would remove "a certain amount of liberty from the individual," and confer "considerable discretionary power on the few," the editor of that journal was opposed to it, "even at the risk of being taken in by a quack, now and then, or continuing to be exposed to the assaults of the germs." [33]

After all the debate within organized homeopathy, the moderates won the day. In 1912 representatives of the A.M.A. and the A.I.H. agreed to co-sponsor a bill to establish a national bureau of health.[34] Unfortunately, opposition was to be so powerful that it was not until 1953 that the Department of Health, Education, and Welfare was founded.

From 1900 to 1920, homeopathic medicine clearly was in decline. The statistics of the homeopathic colleges best demonstrate the losing struggle. The number of schools reached a high of about twenty-two in 1900. Then they began to disappear; by 1923 only two homeopathic medical colleges remained in operation. In 1903 homeopathy had been recognized by the A.M.A., which invited homeopathic graduates to join the ranks of orthodox medicine. By 1920, however, the homeopathic schools which remained in operation were unable to attract enough students. At the same time, the homeopathic sect was being depleted by the deaths of many of the older members.

The decline was caused primarily by revolutionary changes in American medical education which occurred during the progressive era. In 1887 Dr. Frederick H. Gerrish of the Maine Board of Health reported to the American Academy of Medicine that the quality of education was shockingly low. He had an eight-year-old girl send a letter of inquiry to a number of colleges, in an obviously immature handwriting. She admitted her complete ignorance of "natural philosophy" (the study of the physical universe) and the other prerequisites, but she expressed a desire to become a physician. About half of the schools "evinced a willingness to take the fee of the applicant, and promised to make a doctor of her in spite of her confessed

---

[32] *Homeopathic Recorder* 27 (February 1912): 92–93.
[33] Ibid.
[34] *Journal of the American Institute of Homeopathy* 5 (July 1912): 63; (September 1912): 245.

inability to pass the examination." One college wrote: "Our examination is not difficult; no one has yet failed to pass." Another assured her that the tests were designed to insure that "no deserving applicant is rejected on account of not being able to pass them." [35]

Improved education began in 1890 with the formation of the Association of American Medical Colleges. Fifty-five schools sent delegates to its first convention, where they adopted a series of proposals. They required oral and written examinations, established stringent admission standards, and adopted a three-year course of study. By 1893 the A.M.A. was able to report that less than 10 per cent of the colleges maintained the insufficient two-year term, while several of the more forward-looking had extended their course to four years. Moreover, the A.M.A. noted that there was a direct correlation between quality of education and the students' chances of success at the medical boards. Twenty-five per cent of the graduates of the poorer schools were unable to pass the examinations, while over 98 per cent of those from the better colleges passed.[36] In 1895 standards were raised even higher, with the adoption of a four-year course by the association of colleges. The A.M.A. announced that it would no longer admit graduates of schools not meeting the national standards. The result was that every "reputable" northern school soon required a four-year course of medical studies.[37]

Along with the development of higher standards, more and more states adopted medical licensure laws. In 1888 only five states required examinations. By 1896, twenty-three states tested every applicant. Of those, sixteen had a single board of examiners, four had homeopathic and allopathic boards, while the other three maintained allopathic, homeopathic, and eclectic boards.[38] As the various states reported the results of their examinations, it became apparent that graduates of inferior schools were incapable of passing the exams. More than 10 per cent of the graduates of 10 of the 16 homeopathic colleges failed the 1908 boards. Failure, however, was not restricted to the irregulars. Of the 123 allopathic schools, 82 had that same dubious distinction. Interestingly, the figures indicated that a slightly higher percentage of the orthodox schools were inferior.[39]

[35] *New York Times*, September 8, 1887, p. 4, col. 4.
[36] *Journal of the A.M.A.* 14 (June 7, 1890): 829–30; 20 (January 7, 1893): 24.
[37] Ibid. 24 (January 26, 1895): 137–38; 34 (June 16, 1900): 1159.
[38] James R. Parsons, "Preliminary Education, Professional Training, and Practice in New York," *Journal of the A.M.A.* 26 (June 13, 1896): 1149–52.
[39] *Journal of the A.M.A.* 52 (May 22, 1909): 1691ff.

Improved standards of medical education, then, coupled with the licensure legislation to eliminate a number of inadequate schools. These developments proved far more destructive to homeopathy than to the orthodox profession. A greater percentage of the homeopathic colleges disappeared because of their inability to meet the requirements. As noted earlier, only two of the twenty-two colleges remained open in 1923.[40] The development of the single examining board wreaked havoc with the irregular schools. In order to pass the test, all graduates had to be competent in the nonsectarian medical fields; homeopathic *materia medica* and therapeutics were cast into the background. As homeopathy lost ground, graduates from homeopathic schools in the early twentieth century were in many cases "mongrel" allopaths, being homeopaths in name only.

In 1910 medical education received a great boost through the publication of Abraham Flexner's intensive and celebrated examination of the American colleges.[41] His study, sponsored by the Carnegie Foundation, has traditionally been considered the turning point in the development of modern medical schools. It was in effect an attempt to publicize the disgraceful conditions which remained in spite of the advances from 1885 to 1909. Those advances provided a firm basis for Flexner's evaluation, but his work was only one step in a much larger movement. Medical education had improved immeasurably during the early progressive era. The curriculum was expanded, the course of study lengthened, clinical work emphasized, and strict entrance requirements were adopted. Flexner's major role was in evaluating the way the various colleges applied these standards.

In making his study, Flexner did an almost unbelievable amount of work. He tracked down the academic records of hundreds of transfer students, often to discover that failing grades had been accepted for advanced credit by a number of colleges. In other cases, he found that so-called "transfer students" had never enrolled at the college they claimed to have originally attended.[42] In addition, Flexner discovered that a great many colleges required a four-year high school education, but when he inquired he was informed that many of the secondary schools had provided only two or three years of work, and some schools did not exist. Colleges were admitting students who claimed to have graduated from "high schools" which Flexner could not locate, even with the assistance of educa-

[40] Ibid. 43 (August 13, 1904): 466–68; 51 (August 15, 1908): 606–8.

[41] Abraham Flexner, *Medical Education in the United States and Canada* (Boston, 1910).

[42] See for instance the Baltimore Medical College folder in box 18, Abraham Flexner papers, Library of Congress.

tors of the region.[43] Flexner concluded that three-fourths of the medical schools were totally inadequate.

Flexner made no distinction between homeopathic and orthodox schools.[44] But his report publicized the inadequacies of unorthodox education. Fewer students would be enrolling now in the homeopathic colleges, especially since Flexner had proved that graduates of the inferior schools had wasted their time at colleges which could not prepare them for the state boards.

In an editorial in the *Journal of the American Institute of Homeopathy*, Dr. F. E. Ford declared that homeopaths had not advanced since the days of Hahnemann. Over the past century, however, the allopath had "revolutionized his practice." The result was that each medical sect was being judged upon its merits, he said, and that homeopathic schools cannot compete with the orthodox ones. "The A.M.A., while somewhat drastic," he asserted, "is on the right track. There should be uniform standards of medical education, therapeutics excepted."[45] Interestingly, an earlier editorial expressed anger that Flexner was not a trained physician. According to the editor, he was incapable of judging quality medical education. "Let the shoemaker stick to his last," was the indignant advice given to the author of the famous report.[46]

Another analysis of the homeopathic dilemma was provided by the *Homeopathic Recorder*, an organ of the high potency men. The editor asserted that the homeopathic colleges were closing because they "didn't teach pure homeopathy." The schools wasted too much time on anatomy, physiology, surgery, and the other required subjects, while neglecting the study of *materia medica*, which should take precedence in the training of a homeopath. Physicians gave the patients the quick relief of symptoms they demanded by administering the newer miracle drugs. Theoretically, the master homeopathic prescribers of the past would have sought the underlying cause of illness and using homeopathic remedies would have eliminated it.[47]

The *Hahnemannian Monthly*, which also represented the pure home-

[43] Flexner to S. E. Weber, New York City, August 17, 1909; J. J. Dostler to Flexner, University, Alabama, June 12, 1909, MSS in ibid.

[44] *Journal of the American Institute of Homeopathy* 3 (September 1910): 225–27. For the reaction of some of the allopathic schools, see the *Chicago Record-Herald*, June 6, 1910, p. 1, col 7; p. 2, cols. 1–4; June 7, 1910, p. 3, col. 2; p. 8, col. 2. Chicago was hit hard by the Flexner Report, which called the city the "plague spot of the country in Medical Education."

[45] *Journal of the American Institute of Homeopathy* 2 (June 1910): 387–88.

[46] *North American Journal of Homeopathy*, 3d ser., 25 (September 1910): 597–600.

[47] *Homeopathic Recorder* 25 (November 1910): 481–84.

opaths, declared that the new standards were too high. The attempt of the A.M.A. and the Carnegie Foundation to improve medical education, it said, had been carried too far. Two years of college, four of medical school, and one more as an intern, a total of seven years, "would consume too much time and too much money to be within the reach of the average American young man." The magazine believed that the improved standards only strengthened homeopathy's competition. The allopathic school appealed to the well-born, who could afford a seven-year course, while the inferior systems did not abide by the A.M.A. regulations and provided a less expensive medical education. The enemy was being assisted, then, while homeopathy, which traditionally had attracted a number of less affluent students, was faltering.[48]

The more moderate American Institute of Homeopathy committee on medical examining boards reported in 1917 that the decline in homeopathy was caused by an inability to recognize the problem. While so many homeopaths were denouncing the A.M.A., Flexner, and the Carnegie Foundation, the real difficulty was the inadequate education provided by so many of the homeopathic colleges. "We know the requirements," the report continued. "It's up to us to get busy, get behind our schools, and see that they equal, yea, excel the requirements of the best."[49]

At the same time that the Hahnemannians were busily condemning the A.M.A. and the treasonous colleges, and the liberal homeopaths were demanding improved standards, the colleges were either closing their doors or becoming allopathic. In 1909, when enrollment dwindled to a mere three students, the homeopathic department of the University of Minnesota was abolished by vote of the board of regents. Electives remained in homeopathic *materia medica* and therapeutics.[50]

The events in Minnesota were portents of the future. In 1914 the Cleveland-Pulte Medical College closed its doors. Through the influence of the American Institute of Homeopathy, however, Ohio State University opened a homeopathic division in Columbus, which endured only until 1922.[51] In 1915 the Hahnemann College of the Pacific merged with the University of California Medical School at San Francisco. Under the amalgamation plan, all students took the nonsectarian courses together, but *materia medica* and

[48] *Hahnemannian Monthly* 52 (August 1917): 499.

[49] *Journal of the American Institute of Homeopathy* 10 (September 1917): 352-55.

[50] *Journal of the A.M.A.* 52 (May 15, 1909): 1600; *Journal of the American Institute of Homeopathy* 1 (August 1909): 363-64.

[51] *New England Medical Gazette* 49 (June 1914): 335.

therapeutics were taught separately to those intending to practice homeopathy. Although homeopathy was still on the curriculum, one more college had taken the first step toward its obliteration.[52]

The four remaining homeopathic schools were at Boston University, the University of Michigan, the New York Homeopathic Medical College, and Philadelphia's Hahnemann Medical College. The first two were to undergo a complete transformation, resulting in the elimination of homeopathy, while the latter were to remain homeopathic until the 1950's. In the case of Boston University, as early as 1907 the president asked the faculty to inform him as "to the probable future of homeopathy."[53]

While Harvard, Tufts, Columbia, Johns Hopkins, and the other leading orthodox colleges all showed an increased enrollment from 1908 to 1917, Hahnemann Medical College lost 33 per cent of its students, Boston University's enrollment decreased by 40 per cent, Michigan Homeopathic lost 42 per cent, and the only homeopathic college to gain students was the New York Homeopathic, which reported an increase of 113 per cent.[54] On April 30, 1917, in the face of such statistics, Dr. Nelson Wood suggested to the staff of the Massachusetts Homeopathic Hospital that an allopathic chair be established at Boston University.

There was no real change until President L. H. Murlin became disturbed at the decreasing enrollment. He could not understand why applications had fallen off at a time when more students were anticipated. It was expected that the existing schools would be strengthened by the elimination of the weaker ones. Moreover, Murlin had thought that since the allopaths had welcomed homeopaths into their societies, the "new school" certainly would advance. He decided that the problem must result from the fact that homeopathy was sectarian. To many the word "homeopathy" indicated "peculiar, sectarian, and bigoted." Calling for an end to all sectarianism, Murlin advocated a more scientific approach to medical education.[55]

The medical faculty appointed a committee to investigate the proposed reorganization, and it soon reported that a change was necessary for the survival of the school. When the alumni were polled, 75 per cent of those who replied favored the elimination of unorthodox designations. Express-

---

[52] *Journal of the American Institute of Homeopathy* 8 (August 1915): 180–81, 198–200; J. W. Ward to L. C. Boyd, San Francisco, September 8, 1923, MS in Michigan Homeopathic Medical School Papers, Michigan Historical Collections.

[53] *History of the Reorganization of the Boston University School of Medicine* (Boston, 1918), pp. 1–2.

[54] Ibid., pp. 18–19.

[55] Ibid., pp. 2–5.

ing a desire for the advantages of a "regular" diploma, the entire gradua-
ting class of 1918 petitioned for courses in old-school therapeutics. On
June 6, 1918, responding to the widespread demand, Boston University
became an orthodox school. By 1922 the courses in homeopathy had degenerated into a series of lectures combining the history of medicine with
homeopathic *materia medica*.[56]

The homeopathic department of the University of Michigan was next
to disappear. As the "separate institutions entail much unnecessary expense
to the state," the legislature adopted a joint resolution recommending the
consolidation of the homeopathic and allopathic divisions. Many homeopaths recognized that this was wise. In 1921 there were 554 orthodox students, as compared to only 64 homeopathic ones.[57] On the other hand, convinced that amalgamation eventually would lead to the elimination of
homeopathy, the homeopathic faculty opposed any change. First of all, they
argued that the practice of homeopathy presupposed an intensive study of
drug action. This type of education could not be undertaken as a minor
aspect of medical training; under the reorganization plan, sectarian courses
would clearly be considered secondary to the basic medical subjects. Moreover, since the allopaths considered homeopathy to be a delusion, the
faculty declared that any consolidation would be a step toward the destruction of their system.[58]

Dr. Royal Copeland presented the homeopathic case before the regents
on December 9, 1921. He declared that it was ridiculous to attempt to edu-
cate the two sects in the same classes. "You might just as well try to mix
oil and water, to bring [together] the Republican and Democratic parties,
or have a labor union convention in the office of the United States Steel
Corporation. It can't be done." He insisted that instead of seeing homeopathy destroyed by an unwanted merger, he would rather have the regents
disband the homeopathic school.[59] His arguments were disregarded, and
the merger was completed.

At the 1922 meeting of the American Institute of Homeopathy, the
council on medical education presented a report which must have depressed

[56] "Complete Report of the Committee on Reorganization," pp. 1–2, bound in
ibid.
[57] D. W. Springer to President M. L. Burton, March 14, 1921, carbon copy in
Homeopathic Medical School Papers.
[58] "Present Facts about Combination," paper prepared by W. B. Hinsdale,
W. A. Dewey et al., carbon copy in Homeopathic Medical School Papers.
[59] Speech of Royal Copeland, carbon copy, in ibid.; Hinsdale to regents,
January 27, 1922, carbon copy in Hinsdale Papers, Michigan Historical Collections.

every homeopath in attendance. It declared that homeopathic institutions were "in deplorable condition." Boston University had graduated no homeopaths during the past year; Hahnemann of Philadelphia had produced only 17; throughout the nation, there were only 62 homeopathic graduates. By 1923 there were only two homeopathic colleges in existence—New York Homeopathic and Hahnemann of Philadelphia. Homeopathy was disappearing from the American scene.[60]

Stuart Close, a high potency advocate from Brooklyn, in an article on the "Future of Homeopathy," attributed the decline of his system to a number of factors. First, he insisted that the sect had been betrayed by many of its own members, namely those who had belittled Hahnemann and his diligent followers. By openly advocating the unification of the entire medical profession, these "traitors" were rushing homeopathy to its grave. Another reason for the decline of homeopathy, he said, was that few physicians were interested in philosophy, and homeopathy had always attracted those with philosophical leanings. Like a great many of his colleagues, Close urged the establishment of postgraduate schools to teach homeopathy as a specialty. Yet, at the same time, he urged his fellow homeopaths to enter the mainstream of American medicine, which could only mean joining the A.M.A.[61]

In June of 1921 fourteen high potency advocates led by Dr. Julia M. Green organized the American Foundation for Homeopathy. They intended the organization to provide education through postgraduate courses, to inform the public of the benefits of homeopathy, and to serve as a repository for information and literature. Homeopathy had come full circle from its position as a minority in the 1840's, when it was universally condemned by the most prominent allopaths. During the 1880's and 1890's it had become respectable, and in 1903 the A.M.A. even accepted homeopaths as members. Yet, by 1920 homeopathy had witnessed a drastic decline. For the remaining years of the century, homeopathy, with its colleges disappearing and with fewer and fewer graduates, seemed to be heading for total extinction.

[60] *Journal of the American Institute of Homeopathy* 15 (September 1922): 251–53.
[61] Stuart Close, "The Future of Homeopathy," *Hahnemannian Monthly* 61 (September 1921): 561–74.

XII

THE SEARCH FOR SALVATION

THE ORGANIZATION OF THE American Foundation for Homeopathy was the first meaningful action intended to prevent the disappearance of the sect. The Foundation's postgraduate course, however, was almost a total failure. Although it has continued into the 1960's, it introduced relatively few physicians to homeopathy. It certainly could not take the place of the extinct medical colleges. Over a period of more than forty years, it seems evident that less than one hundred and fifty doctors attended the course. Moreover, many of those enrolling were foreigners who had no intention of practicing in the United States. When it became obvious that few orthodox practitioners were interested in becoming homeopaths, the trustees of the Foundation voted to admit osteopaths, dentists, and veterinarians. Despite its long struggle to maintain its course, the Foundation has been unable to train enough physicians to guarantee the continued existence of homeopathy.[1] Even the formation of "layman's leagues" in various cities, which were expected to encourage a demand for more and better homeopathic care, could not succeed without an adequate supply of homeopathic physicians.

While the postgraduate course was operating at a monetary loss, the high potency advocates who had sponsored it were becoming increasingly

---

[1] Much of the material in this chapter is highly interpretive, based upon reading in twentieth century homeopathic medical journals, a series of oral history interviews with leading homeopaths (under the auspices of the National Library of Medicine), and manuscript material located in the files of the American Foundation for Homeopathy, Washington, D.C. Unfortunately, the Foundation was reluctant to allow the author to quote from its files, due to the fact that many of the letters mentioned individuals still alive in 1970.

disgusted with the quality of education at the two homeopathic colleges. Moreover, the Hahnemannians recognized that it was almost impossible for a sect as small as homeopathy to support good medical schools. In the first place, the twentieth century emphasis on laboratory and clinical work necessitated the construction of elaborate and expensive facilities. Moreover, with the development of unified examining boards, homeopathic courses were relegated to a minor role in the curriculum. The instruction in homeopathy was given short shrift in favor of the subjects required for licensure. Obviously, the homeopathic colleges could not compete with colleges having large endowments and enough resources to pay high salaries and purchase the latest instruments.

Interestingly, the recognition that homeopathy was being poorly taught at the colleges reinforced the need for the Foundation, in spite of its inadequacies. With the dearth of homeopathic instruction, there was no alternative. The postgraduate course had to produce competent homeopaths, or homeopathy would soon disappear from the American scene.

For a number of reasons, however, the members of the American Institute of Homeopathy refused to work with the Foundation. While the Foundation sought to expand the role of the patient, many physicians were angered at the implication that laymen would determine the future of homeopathy. In addition, while advertising was traditionally considered unethical, a major goal of the Foundation was to publicize the benefits of homeopathy. Finally, the old conflict between high and low potency discouraged closer relations between the Institute and the Foundation. The extravagant claims of the Hahnemannians had always been embarrassing to the more "eclectic" homeopaths who controlled the A.I.H., yet the Foundation had been organized by high potency advocates. The net result was that the members of the Institute considered the Foundation an instrument of the conservative wing of homeopathy.

While the high potency men were outraged at the inadequate homeopathic instruction, the Institute was satisfied that the two colleges (Hahnemann of Philadelphia and the New York Homeopathic) received class A ratings by the A.M.A. Toward the end of the 1920's, the A.I.H. voted to establish a college around the nucleus of Cleveland's Huron Road Hospital. At the same time, Chicago's homeopathic practitioners initiated a drive to endow a school in that city.[2] The advent of the Great Depression, however, prevented the completion of those plans, and when it became impossible

---

[2] *Journal of the American Institute of Homeopathy* 21 (August 1928): 642.

to raise funds, the proposals were dropped.[3] This conflict within the homeopathic ranks prevented the unity necessary to preserve homeopathy. While the Institute homeopaths were attempting to increase the number of colleges, the Hahnemannians were bitterly denouncing the quality of education at the existing schools.

In 1924 Dr. Morris Fishbein, associate editor of the *Journal of the American Medical Association*, began to write books and articles critical of homeopathy. He upset a great many followers of Hahnemann when he referred to homeopathy in a book entitled *Medical Follies*.[4] He also described the "Rise and Fall of Homeopathy" in a popular magazine. Rather surprisingly, in the latter, Fishbein declared that Hahnemann's influence had been beneficial. The German theorist, he said, had demonstrated that small doses were superior to larger ones, and that patients must be handled on an individual basis. After complimenting homeopathy, Fishbein showed statistically that the sect had definitely declined, and he predicted that it would soon disappear from the American scene.[5]

He attributed its fall to several factors. First, he asserted that while scientific medicine was advancing, homeopathy remained tied to an exclusive and dogmatic theory. This meant that homeopathy was becoming increasingly inferior to orthodox practice. In consequence, the modern homeopath was losing confidence in his system, and thus, many homeopathic graduates were converting to allopathic medicine. In the second place, Fishbein said, the internal divisions which affected homeopathy played a major role in destroying the system. When unity was most needed, it could not be achieved. Finally, he pointed out that homeopathy could not finance adequate medical schools in a time of spiralling costs. He concluded by declaring that the "history of homeopathy is distinct and peculiar. It records the propounding and acceptance of a theory which, in itself wrong, nevertheless influenced the steps of a beginning science into paths that were right."[6]

Dr. Stuart Close, a prominent Hahnemannian, responded to Fishbein in an issue of the *Homeopathic Recorder*. He admitted that Fishbein had "brought to light and given publicity to some undeniable facts about the present status of the homeopathic organization." Close, however, took ex-

---

[3] Ibid. 27 (November 1934): 680–84.
[4] Morris Fishbein, *Medical Follies* (New York, 1925), pp. 29–43.
[5] Morris Fishbein, "The Rise and Fall of Homeopathy," *American Mercury* 2 (June 1924): 150–54.
[6] Ibid.

ception to the implication that the fall of homeopathy was at all related to its inadequacy and inefficiency. He insisted that its weakness stemmed from the fact that its organizations were "too much occupied with personalities, politics, wire-pulling and many other things which have nothing to do with homeopathy." The "physical organism of homeopathy, the institution," he said, "is dying, or rather it is in a state of transition." While the sect may disappear, its "spirit" and its "truths" would always remain.[7]

Close may well have been correct in his belief that homeopathy had not declined as a result of its lack of success. Practicing homeopaths seemed to be thriving, and most of them were quite familiar with the allopathic advances of the day. Daniel E. S. Coleman, another homeopath, agreed with Close that the disappearance of the schools did not result from any failure of homeopathic theory. Rather, the schools closed due to a *"financial inability to meet the requirements."* If homeopathic inadequacy had destroyed the colleges, one would expect more homeopathic than allopathic schools to have vanished. Yet, from 1901 to 1925, seventeen homeopathic and fifty-three allopathic colleges had closed their doors. Orthodox colleges as well as irregular ones had difficulty in maintaining the steadily improving standards and in meeting the increasing cost of medical education.[8]

Late in 1935 the A.M.A. council on medical education and hospitals added to the many problems of organized homeopathy when it resolved that after July 1, 1938, the approved list of schools and hospitals would not include institutions of "sectarian medicine." The orthodox physicians argued quite convincingly that "the advance of the medical sciences have been and should be independent of any sectarian point of view, and [that] medical education should not be handicapped or directed by a dogmatic attitude towards disease." Homeopathic institutions would have to abandon their sectarianism, as well as their names.[9] A storm of outraged indignation swept through the homeopathic world. Homeopathic societies were bitter in their denunciation of the intolerant attitude of the allopathic profession.[10]

Although the homeopathic organizations were quick to condemn the A.M.A. for what they felt was its renewed evidence of bigotry, a number

[7] Stuart Close, "The Present Status of Homeopathy as viewed by an associate editor of the J.A.M.A.," *Homeopathic Recorder* 39 (September 1924): 409–17; (October 1924): 459–66.
[8] Daniel E. S. Coleman, "The Follies of Doctor Fishbein," *Journal of the American Institute of Homeopathy* 19 (February 1926): 110–21.
[9] *Journal of the A.M.A.* 105 (October 5, 1935): 1123.
[10] *Journal of the American Institute of Homeopathy* 29 (January 1936): 44–45.

of homeopaths had come to the conclusion that the term "homeopathy" was indeed detrimental to their progress. Since the days of Egbert Guernsey, some homeopaths had been arguing for the elimination of the title. In 1924 the editor of the *Homeopathic Recorder*, Dr. Rudolph F. Rabe, proposed that the sectarian name be abandoned. Homeopathic research, he said, not only had accomplished nothing since the nineteenth century, but homeopaths were notorious for their failure to keep up with the medical advances of the day. He hoped that the doctrines of homeopathy might be preserved under a new label, and the trend of the day reversed.[11]

Since a change in name had been advocated by a number of respected physicians, the college administrators had an excellent excuse for acceding to the demands of the A.M.A. Moreover, it was generally recognized that any school taken off the approved list would be destroyed by an inability to attract students. Graduates of an unapproved school would not receive the choice hospital appointments and thus might be denied the opportunity for professional advancement.

On February 16, 1936 Dean Claude A. Burrett reported that more than one-half of the alumni of the New York Homeopathic Medical College were in favor of renaming the school the "New York Medical College." Recognizing that survival was at stake, the board of trustees decided to make the change. Burrett explained to the American Institute of Homeopathy that the A.M.A. council on medical education was responsible. A school rated less than class A could not guarantee success at the state examining boards, and so it could not hope to enroll top-flight students. Burrett noted that the college now would be able to attract excellent medical educators and students, while homeopathy would still be taught.[12]

The year after the A.M.A. had used its power to force the homeopathic institutions to eliminate the word "homeopathic" from their names, the fear of socialized medicine encouraged the establishment of a closer relationship between homeopathy and the orthodox profession. To the American physician, the New Deal was a giant step toward regimentation. As soon as the Sheppard Towner Maternal and Infant Protection Act was proposed in 1920, the A.M.A. was up in arms against the threat of "state medicine." When the Social Security Act was passed in 1935, the profession grew more wary of "incursions" upon American liberty.[13]

---

[11] *Homeopathic Recorder* 39 (March 1924): 97–105.
[12] *Journal of the American Institute of Homeopathy* 29 (April 1936): 251–52.
[13] See James Burrow, *A.M.A.: Voice of American Medicine* (Baltimore, 1963), pp. 161–64, 194ff.

Ohio's Dr. Lucy Stone Herzog, a homeopath who recognized the "threat," became the leader of an attempt to work with the A.M.A. in opposing all such legislation. From 1937 to 1940 almost every issue of the *Journal of the American Institute of Homeopathy* included an article by Herzog condemning the "un-American" tendencies of the Roosevelt years. She urged her colleagues to cast aside their caution and to work with the A.M.A., which she called the "savior of American medicine." She insisted that in order to prevent the socialization of medical care, every physician had to support the A.M.A.[14]

Through the influence of Herzog, the A.I.H. established a committee to co-operate with the orthodox association.[15] In 1940 she reported that "the homeopathic school has joined the dominant school in a united front for the duration of the war against regimentation of the medical profession and to prevent socialized medicine." She warned the allopaths not to reward their homeopathic allies by returning to the intolerance of the past. "If we help to accomplish these objectives, the homeopaths do not want to find their ally of the firing line ready to stick a dirk under the ribs, with plans drawn to absorb, destroy, or eliminate them as a medical entity." Herzog calmed the more reluctant Hahnemannians by asserting that it would be foolish for the A.M.A. to attack its homeopathic friends. Two political action groups were certainly more effective than one.[16]

The unity of the depression years apparently convinced a number of homeopaths that the orthodox profession was ready to accept the followers of Hahnemann on an equal basis. A movement was initiated to make homeopathy a therapeutic specialty, rather than continuing to pretend that it was a completely independent system of medical practice. As early as 1944 Rabe suggested that sectarianism would disappear if such a change occurred.[17] Two years later, at a meeting of the A.I.H. congress of states, two distinct proposals were discussed. One group of homeopaths favored the adoption of a nonsectarian name, "homeotherapy." Another group wanted their sect to become a specialty in therapeutics.[18]

[14] See, for instance, *Journal of the American Institute of Homeopathy* 30 (December 1937): 738–49; Lucy Stone Herzog, "A Resume of the Special Session of the House of Delegates at Chicago," *Journal of the American Institute of Homeopathy* 31 (December 1938): 736–41.

[15] *Journal of the American Institute of Homeopathy* 32 (February 1939): 89; (May 1939): 296–302.

[16] Ibid. 33 (March 1940): 157ff.

[17] Ibid. 37 (February 1944): 35–36; 39 (March 1946): 80–81.

[18] Ibid. 39 (April 1946): 26.

In 1950 a committee was appointed to investigate the possibility of forming a specialty board and securing recognition from the A.M.A. The committee consisted of four leading homeopaths. The chairman was G. Kent Smith, a young Californian who was the driving force behind the proposal. Elizabeth Wright Hubbard, the respected and successful New York Hahnemannian, was also on the committee. Joining Smith and Hubbard were Julia M. Green, the head of the Foundation, and a West Coast homeopath of some distinction, Allen C. Neiswander.[19] After considerable soul-searching, the committee decided that they should strive for the acceptance of homeopathy as a specialty within the orthodox school. Basing their requirements for admission on those of the American Board of Internal Medicine, the committee established plans for a homeopathic board. They hoped that they could receive sanction from the A.M.A.; at that point, homeopathy would have been saved by its new-found acceptability.

At the 1953 A.I.H. convention, Green, Smith, and Hubbard insisted in the majority report that homeopathy "is still superior to other forms of medicine." It was essential, however, that "its presentation to the medical profession must be dressed up in suitable clothes so that the younger doctors will take notice." They said that the first thing to do was to shed the "sectarian garb and dress it up as a specialty where it belongs." The report noted that the A.M.A. advisory board for medical specialties had recommended the incorporation of a homeopathic board as a specialty under the American Institute of Homeopathy. When the program was perfected, the homeopaths would apply for recognition. Presumably, homeopathy would become an accepted medical specialty, and sanction by the A.M.A. would preserve the foundering sect.

Although most homeopaths recognized that they had to do something to save their sect from extinction, a few of them opposed the drive to make homeopathy a specialty. Dr. Lewis P. Crutcher, for instance, who earlier had joined the League for Medical Freedom, declared that the attempt to gain acceptance by the A.M.A. was "cowardly." That drive, he exclaimed, was similar to the suggestion that "Protestantism become a 'specialty' under the control of the Roman Catholic Church . . . or . . . that the Republican Party remedy its embarrassment by knuckling as a 'specialty' to the mastery of the numerically stronger Democratic Party." Crutcher was furious at his colleagues. How could they let their group "swallow its pride," "garb it-

[19] For more information on this attempt, see the files of the *Journal of the American Institute of Homeopathy* and the *Homeopathic Recorder*, for 1950–53.

THE SEARCH FOR SALVATION

self" in the "ignominious sackcloth and ashes," and beg its old enemy for mercy?[20]

Although nothing came of the earlier movement for specialty status, the homeopaths continued working for its sanction. During the late 1950's Dr. Wyrth Post Baker, a young homeopath from the District of Columbia, took up the fight. "It is time to divest ourselves of any paranoid delusions of persecution by the A.M.A.," he said. Although orthodox medicine had been wrong in the past, "the life of homeopathy and our individual liberties will be lost unless we support our colleagues in their fight for the survival of private medical practice."[21] Despite the early failure, Baker still seemed to believe that the A.M.A. might recognize homeopathy as a specialty within organized medicine.

During the 1960's, Baker's hopes were realized to some extent. In 1960 the International Hahnemannian Association cast aside all the bitterness of the high and low potency fight and voted itself out of existence. Since by that time almost every Hahnemannian was a member of the Institute, the latter body became the spokesman for organized homeopathy. The *Journal of the American Institute of Homeopathy* absorbed the *Homeopathic Recorder*, the organ of the International Association. Homeopaths finally seemed to recognize that without unity, the death of their sect was imminent. The American Board of Homeotherapeutics was established by Henry Eisfelder of New York, in the hope of becoming recognized as a specialty board. Despite the unprecedented homeopathic unity, the A.M.A. continued to refuse to accept it as a branch of orthodox medicine. The allopaths were willing to consider homeopathy a specialty under the A.I.H., but not, as the homeopaths were requesting, a subspecialty under the heading of "internal medicine."

While many homeopaths were devoting energy and hard work to the fruitless drive to make their practice a specialty, several other attempts to save homeopathy were occurring. In 1950, largely as a result of the enthusiasm of Dr. Chal Bryant of Seattle, the A.I.H. began to raise funds to lobby for the teaching of homeopathy in the various state medical colleges. Bryant concentrated his early efforts on the newly established University of Washington Medical School. Beginning in February of 1951 he proposed that the legislature establish a homeopathic department. According to his plan, every student would be required to take a course in homeopathy. The

[20] *Journal of the American Institute of Homeopathy* 44 (January 1951): 11–15.
[21] Wyrth Post Baker, "The Place of Homeopathy in American Medicine," *Journal of the American Institute of Homeopathy* 50 (November–December 1957): 296–98.

death of Bryant, however, brought this movement to a halt. He seemed to have been the only homeopath who considered the objective within the realm of possibility. When he died, no one stepped forward to take up the cause.[22]

In 1967 Dr. William W. Young, a dynamic practitioner from Chillicothe, Ohio, proposed what he called the "Perpetuation and Propagation Program." According to the P.P.P., the homeopaths would use their funds to establish a series of lectureships. Prominent scientists would be hired to speak on comparative pharmaco-therapeutics. Although this program could hardly save homeopathy, it might preserve the homeopathic doctrines. When he was elected president of the A.I.H. in 1967 by the "young rebels" whose "voices have been ignored too long," the "Perpetuation and Propagation Program" became a distinct possibility.[23] It remains to be seen whether homeopaths will be able to convince leading scientists to accept the offer.

Homeopathy not only had to fight to preserve its existence but it also had to protect itself from infiltration by unqualified practitioners. During the 1950's several chiropractors established so called "homeopathic colleges" in the hope of producing respectable and licensed physicians. Those schools were no more than diploma mills. The most notorious was Fremont University in Los Angeles. It was founded by Joe Hough, who soon was making arrangements to license his graduates in Maryland, where Robert Reddick, the superintendent of a state hospital, had assumed control of the defunct homeopathic licensing board. Reddick issued licenses to several hundred drugless healers, who claimed to be homeopathic practitioners.

When the A.M.A. learned of the scandalous situation, it quickly informed the American Institute of Homeopathy and the legitimate members of the Maryland board, who were innocent of all wrongdoing. An injunction was issued prohibiting the examination of unqualified applicants. In addition, all licenses previously issued were declared to be null and void. In 1957 Reddick was sentenced to four years in the Maryland penitentiary for having back-dated a medical license for a garage mechanic. Homeopaths

---

[22] Carl H. Enstam, "Post-Graduate Homeopathic Education on the Pacific Coast," *Journal of the American Institute of Homeopathy* 40 (May 1957): 167–68; Chal Bryant, "An Appeal with a Definite Program for the Establishment and Perpetuation of Homeopathic Instruction in the Universities of the United States," *Journal of the American Institute of Homeopathy* 44 (January 1951): 14–15.

[23] W. W. Young, "The Perpetuation and Propagation Program," *Journal of the American Institute of Homeopathy* 60 (July–August 1967): 198–206; (May–June 1967): 138.

reacted quite admirably to a potentially dangerous problem. As soon as they learned of the affair, they took strong action in coordination with the A.M.A.[24]

Despite the best efforts of the homeopaths, the existence of homeopathy is still in jeopardy. By the 1960's, with a few notable exceptions, the average homeopath was well over sixty years old. Every year, death further depletes the ranks. With only a few converts, the future looks grim indeed. Unless the trend can be reversed, homeopathy will not survive more than two or three decades.

The experience of Dr. Allen D. Sutherland of Brattleboro, Vermont will be faced by virtually every one of his homeopathic colleagues. In 1947 he reported that homeopathy in Vermont was at a "low ebb," and that there were only eight practicing homeopaths in his state. "With the exception of the speaker, these are all old men whose lease on life is fast running out."[25] By 1963 the directory of homeopathic physicians listed Dr. Sutherland as the only practitioner in the state of Vermont.[26]

The decline of homeopathy can be attributed to a number of factors. First, while the orthodox profession experienced a series of revolutionary changes which improved their practice, homeopathy remained relatively stagnant. Second, the rapidly rising standards of medical education further threatened the survival of the irregulars. In the third place, in an age of conformity, sectarianism is frowned upon, and a diploma from a regular school became far more valuable than one from a homeopathic college. Finally, in the days of specialism, most graduates of homeopathic colleges became experts in other fields (surgery, ophthalmology, pediatrics, gynecology, and so forth), and in so doing lost their homeopathic heritage.

The tendencies of the times further weakened homeopathy. As Americans became more materialistic, strength was drawn away from the more philosophical and theoretical homeopathy. Students no longer went to medical school to learn theory and philosophy. They wanted to learn pragmatic medicine. As a result, they concentrate upon the required subjects, and give homeopathy no more than a glance. Moreover, the desire and need to in-

---

[24] *Journal of the American Institute of Homeopathy* 46 (December 1953): 371–72; the American Institute of Homeopathy files, maintained temporarily in the attic of Boericke and Tafel drug house, Philadelphia, includes many letters throwing light on the subject; the story was confirmed in a letter from Oliver Field, of the A.M.A. department of investigation, to the author, Chicago, June 19, 1968.

[25] *Journal of the American Institute of Homeopathy* 40 (June 1947): 194.

[26] American Institute of Homeopathy, *1963 Directory* (Philadelphia, 1963), p. 59.

crease efficiency and handle larger patient loads made it necessary for homeopaths to practice allopathically; homeopathy was difficult for the physician to practice, and the results came too slowly to satisfy the average patient. With the greater demand for medical services, the average physician could not spend enough time with his patient, nor did he want to devote hours to taking complete medical histories. Rather, he was forced to prescribe a quick remedy and get on to the next patient.

During the days of apprenticeship, the homeopathic student had worked for several years with his preceptor, and most had prior experience with the system, either through a homeopathic father, a homeopathic family physician, or an intensely philosophical background.[27] To remain an unorthodox practitioner, the physician had to be something of an individualist. As a result, homeopathic organizations were notoriously filled with dissension, back-biting, and internecine warfare. When unity was most needed, during the period from 1900 to 1920, the homeopathic profession was divided into high and low potency wings, each of which wanted nothing to do with the other. It is doubtful, however, that unification would have been able to prevent the rapid decline of the sect.

One can easily see a definite parallel between the history of homeopathy and that of osteopathy, the largest unorthodox sect of the twentieth century. At first, osteopaths were bitterly condemned by the orthodox (and homeopathic) physicians.[28] Graduates of osteopathic schools were looked down upon as semi-professionals, just as homeopaths had been considered second-class physicians during the period from 1840 to 1903. Slowly the orthodox attitude began to change. Colleges of osteopathy raised their standards and strengthened their requirements. In the 1950's osteopaths began to be accepted as physicians by allopaths. In 1967 the A.M.A. house of delegates was authorized to negotiate the conversion of schools of osteopathy to orthodox colleges. As with homeopathy, merger was not effected immediately. The American Osteopathic Association, representing some 16,000 practitioners, wanted to remain as a separate entity. It refused to vote itself out of existence. It condemned those physicians who favored a merger with the much larger and more powerful A.M.A.[29]

Dr. Roy S. Young, the president of the American Osteopathic Associa-

---

[27] Marcia Moore and James Stephenson, "A Motivational and Sociological Analysis of Homeopathic Physicians in the U.S.A. and U.K.," *British Homeopathic Journal* 51 (October 1962): 297–303.

[28] *New York Times*, January 30, 1902, p. 5, col. 5.

[29] See ibid., December 1, 1968, p. 82, cols. 4–5.

tion, echoed the Hahnemannians when he told an audience in 1969 that the A.M.A. intended to destroy osteopathy by inviting it into orthodox medicine.[30] If the osteopaths continue to reject offers to merge with the A.M.A., one can expect that the osteopaths will probably decline in numbers as more and more graduates of their colleges seek to advance in professional status by joining the A.M.A. Those who remain loyal to osteopathy, and attempt to maintain their separate identity, will find themselves fighting a losing battle.

[30] *Boston Globe*, March 10, 1969, p. 21, col. 5.

BIBLIOGRAPHY

I. Primary Sources

A. *Private Papers and Manuscripts*

American Foundation for Homeopathy. Washington, D.C. The files of the Foundation include the Chairman's Reports, 1924–1960, the Reports of the Bureau of Instruction, 1925–1960, the original Statement of Intentions of June, 1921, and a carbon copy of the Report of the Committee to investigate the Idea of Organizing a Specialty in Homeopathy, 1953.

American Institute of Homeopathy. The files of the Institute, which were temporarily located in the attic of Boericke and Tafel druggists, Philadelphia, are being transferred to the Foundation's office in Washington, D.C. They include numerous letters relating to the recent history of homeopathy, but after a few days of research, the author was not allowed to continue with his examination of the material.

American Medical Association. Chicago, Illinois. The A.M.A. archives include nothing prior to the 1920's, and so were useless for this study.

James Angell Papers. Michigan Historical Collections. Ann Arbor, Michigan.

Henry Ingersoll Bowditch Papers. Countway Library. Harvard University. These papers include a number of valuable letters, as well as drafts of unpublished essays on the new code controversy. One important item was the annotated copy of the *Letter of A. Y. P. Garnett, in Reply to Henry I. Bowditch, November, 1887* (Washington, D.C., 1887).

C. M. Bull Papers. Burton Historical Collection. Detroit Public Library.

Chicago Medical Society. Minutes, 1850's and 1860's. These ledgers are located in the Chicago Historical Society. The first volume includes a Brief History of Medical Societies in Chicago, written by N. S. Davis.

Dreer Collection. Historical Society of Pennsylvania. Philadelphia.

Abraham Flexner Papers. Library of Congress. Washington, D.C.

John W. Francis Papers. New York Public Library.

James Garfield Letter Book. Library of Congress. Washington, D.C.

Gratz Collection. Historical Society of Pennsylvania. Philadelphia.

Hamilton County Medical Club. Minutes, 1842–1850. National Library of Medicine. Bethesda, Maryland.

Wilbert Hinsdale Papers. Michigan Historical Collections. Ann Arbor, Michigan.

International Hahnemannian Association. List of Members, 1881. This is located in the library of the Hahnemann Medical College. Philadelphia, Pennsylvania.

Letter from Oliver Field to the author, Chicago, June 19, 1968.

Letter from Orson Fox to C. W. Chidester, Ann Arbor, October 12, 1875. Michigan Historical Collections. Ann Arbor, Michigan.

Letter from Peter Middleton to Charles Clinton, New York City, October 31, 1753. Chicago Historical Society.

John T. Mason Papers. Burton Historical Collection. Detroit Public Library.

Massachusetts Medical Society. Boston, Massachusetts. The files of the Society include two handwritten ledgers, entitled Records of Boards of Trial, 1858–1881, and Records of Boards of Trial, since 1882.

Michigan Homeopathic Medical School Papers. Michigan Historical Collections. Ann Arbor, Michigan.

New York Academy of Medicine. Committee of Ethics. Minutes, September 30, 1867. This is located in a scrapbook housed at the Academy.

William Prescott Papers. New York Public Library.

A. I. Sawyer Papers. Michigan Historical Collections. Ann Arbor, Michigan. Besides innumerable letters, this important collection includes a multi-volume diary, a manuscript History of Homeopathy in Michigan, and notes on Factions in Homeopathy.

Joseph Toner Collection. Library of Congress. Washington, D.C. This gigantic collection includes letters, drafts of essays, and Toner's collection of manuscript material. One valuable item is a volume of lecture notes taken by Alexander Clendinen from the lectures of Benjamin Rush in 1798.

Peter Turner Papers. Library of Congress. Washington, D.C.

University of Michigan Medical Faculty. Minutes, 1850–1875, 1878–1886. Michigan Historical Collections. Ann Arbor, Michigan. Unfortunately, the minutes for the crucial period from 1875 to 1877 are missing.

Edward C. Walker Papers. Michigan Historical Collections. Ann Arbor, Michigan.

Wayne State University Archives. Detroit, Michigan. Scrapbook Number One is valuable for its many clippings on medicine in Michigan, especially relating to education.

William Woodbridge Papers. Burton Historical Collection. Detroit Public Library.

B. *Official Records and Documents*

American Institute of Homeopathy. *Transactions.* 1846–1872.

American Medical Association. *Transactions.* 1848–1882.

City of Boston. Document Number 40. *Proceedings at the Dedication of the City Hospital, May 24, 1864.* Boston: 1864.
———. *Report on the Introduction of Homeopathy into the City Hospital.* Boston: 1864.
City of Chicago. Board of Health. *Report, 1867, 1868 and 1869, and a Sanitary History of Chicago from 1833 to 1870.* Chicago: 1871.
Cook County Board of Commissioners. *Proceedings, 1881–1882.* Chicago: n.d.
Cook County Hospital. *Annual Report, 1884.* Chicago: 1885.
———. *Annual Report, 1887.* Chicago: 1888.
Massachusetts Homeopathic Medical Society. *Publications, 1840–1861.* Taunton: 1871.
———. *Publications, 1871–1877.* Boston: 1878.
Massachusetts Medical Society. *Medical Communications.* Vol. XI, 1874.
———. *Report of a Committee on Homeopathy.* n.p.: 1850.
Medical Society of the County of New York. *Minutes, 1806–1878.* New York: 1880.
Medical Society of the State of New York. *Transactions, 1882–1884.*
Michigan Senate Journal. 1873.
Michigan State Medical Society. *Proceedings, 1867–68.* Detroit: 1869.
———. *Transactions, 1869–1878.*
New York City. Department of Public Charities. Committee of the Board of Governors of the Alms House Department. *Majority and Minority Reports of the Select Committee of the Board of Governors, to whom was referred the subject of introducing Homeopathy into Bellevue Hospital, Submitted January 19, 1858.* Brooklyn: 1858.
New York State Medical Association. *Transactions, 1885.* Albany: 1885.
Ohio State Medical Society. *Transactions of the Twentieth Annual Meeting.* Cincinnati: 1865.
Proceedings of the National Medical Conventions Held in New York, May, 1846, and in Philadelphia, May, 1847. Philadelphia: 1847.
U.S. Commissioner of Pensions. *Report, 1872.* Washington, D.C.: 1872.
U.S. *Congressional Globe.* 37th Cong., 2nd Sess., 1862.
———. 41st Cong., 3rd Sess., 1870–1871.
U.S. Senate. *Report Number 29.* 41st Cong., 2nd Sess., 1870.
University of Michigan. *Proceedings of the Regents, 1837–1864.* Ann Arbor: 1915.
———. *Proceedings of the Regents, 1864–1869.* Ann Arbor: 1870.
———. *Proceedings of the Regents, 1870–1876.* Ann Arbor: 1877.
———. *Proceedings of the Regents, 1891–1896.* Ann Arbor: 1897.

C. Newspapers

Adrian (Michigan) *Daily Times.* 1875.
Boston Evening Transcript. 1870–73.
Boston Evening Traveller. 1871.
Boston Globe. 1869–73, 1969.

Boston Journal. 1870–71.
Boston Post. 1871–73.
Chicago Herald. 1881.
Chicago Record-Herald. 1910–11.
Cleveland Daily True Democrat. 1849.
Daily Inter Ocean (Chicago). 1881.
Detroit Evening News. 1878–83.
Michigan Argus (Ann Arbor). 1868–78.
Michigan Farmer. 1876.
New York Daily Tribune. 1875–1901.
New York Times. 1862–1907.

D. *Periodicals*

American Homeopath. Vol. 10. 1884.
American Homeopathic Observer. Vol. 3. 1866.
American Journal of the Medical Sciences. Vol. 7. 1830.
American Medical Times. Vols. 3–4. 1861–62.
American Mercury. Vol. 2. 1924.
Boston Medical and Surgical Journal. Vols. 24–88. 1841–73.
British Medical Journal. 1881.
Bulletin of the American Academy of Medicine. Vol. 1. 1894.
California Eclectic Medical Journal. Vols. 3–4. 1910–11.
Chicago Medical Examiner. Vol. 12. 1871.
Christian Examiner. Vol. 32. 1842.
Collier's Weekly Magazine. Vol. 47. 1911.
Detroit Review of Medicine and Pharmacy. Vols. 10–11. 1875–76.
Hahnemannian Monthly. Vols. 6–56. 1871–1921.
Homeopathic Recorder. Vols. 24–37. 1909–24.
Homeopathic Times. Vols. 5–6. 1877–79.
Journal of the American Institute of Homeopathy. Vols. 1–60. 1909–67.
Journal of the American Medical Association. Vols. 1–60. 1883–1913.
Maryland Medical Journal. Vol. 47. 1904.
Medical and Surgical Reporter. Vols. 24–29. 1871–73.
Medical Century. Vol. 2. 1894.
Medical Investigator. Vol. 10. 1873.
Medical News. Vol. 55. 1889.
Medical Record. Vol. 71. 1907.
Medical Tribune. Vol. 3. 1881.
Medical Union. Vols. 1–2. 1873–74.
Michigan Medical News. Vol. 4. 1881–82.
Nation. Vol. 36. 1883.
National Eclectic Medical Association Quarterly. Vol. 3. 1911.
New England Medical Gazette. Vols. 6–49. 1871–1914.
New York Journal of Medicine and Surgery. Vol. 2. 1840.
New York Medical Eclectic. Vol. 8. 1881.

New York Medical Journal. Vols. 38–78. 1883–1903.

New York Medical Times. Vols. 10–17. 1880–90.

North American Journal of Homeopathy. Vols. 1–3rd ser., 25. 1851–1910.

North American Review. Vols. 32, 134. 1831, 1882.

Ohio Medical and Surgical Journal. Vol. 1. 1848.

Peninsular and Independent Medical Journal. Vol. 1. 1858.

Peninsular Journal of Medicine. Vol. 11. 1875.

The Scalpel. Vol. 1. 1849.

Select Journal. Vol. 3. 1834.

United States Magazine, and Democratic Review. Vol. 22. 1848.

Western Homeopathic Observer. Vol. 2. 1865.

E. *Books and Pamphlets*

American Institute of Homeopathy. *1963 Directory.* Philadelphia: 1963.

Bayard, E. *Homeopathia and nature against allopathia and art.* New York: 1858.

Beck, John B. *Lectures on Materia Medica and Therapeutics.* New York: 1856.

Bellows, Albert J. *A Memorial to the Trustees of the Free City Hospital, with Statistics and facts, showing the comparative merits of Homeopathy and Allopathy, as shown by Treatment in European Hospitals.* Boston: 1863.

Biddle, John B. *Materia Medica for the use of Students.* 8th ed. Philadelphia: 1878.

Bigelow, Jacob. *Nature in Disease.* Boston: 1854.

Blachford, Thomas W. *Homeopathy Illustrated; An Address Delivered before the Rensselaer County Medical Society.* Albany: 1851.

Bowditch, Henry I. *The Past, Present, and Future Treatment of Homeopathy, Eclecticism, and Kindred Delusions.* Boston: 1887.

———. *Venesection, its abuse formerly—its neglect at the present day.* Boston: 1872.

Bryant, William Cullen. *Popular Considerations on Homeopathy.* New York: 1841.

Buchan, William. *Domestic Medicine, or the Family Physician.* Edinburgh: 1769.

Code of Ethics of the American Medical Association, adopted May, 1847. Philadelphia: 1848.

Cullen, William. *First Lines of the Practice of Physic.* New York: 1801.

Davis, Nathan Smith, *History of the American Medical Association, from its Organization up to January, 1855.* Philadelphia: 1855.

Dewees, William P. *A Practice of Physic.* 2nd ed. Philadelphia: 1833.

Dunglison, Robley. *On Certain Medical Delusions.* Philadelphia: 1842.

Dunster, Edward. *An Argument made before the American Medical Association at Atlanta, May 7, 1879, against the proposed amendment to the code of ethics restricting the teaching of students of irregular or exclusive systems of medicine.* Ann Arbor: 1879.

Eberle, John. *A Treatise on the Practice of Medicine.* Philadelphia: 1845.

Ewell, James. *Medical Companion, or Family Physician.* 3rd ed. Philadelphia: 1816.

——. *Planter's and Mariner's Medical Companion.* Philadelphia: 1807.

Fishbein, Morris. *Medical Follies.* New York: 1925.

Flexner, Abraham. *Medical Education in the United States and Canada.* Boston: 1910.

Flint, Austin. *A Treatise on the Principles and Practice of Medicine.* Philadelphia: 1866.

Hahnemann, Samuel. *The Chronic Diseases.* New York: 1846.

——. *Lesser Writings.* Edited by R. E. Dudgeon. New York: 1852.

——. *Materia Medica Pura.* Translated by R. E. Dudgeon. London: 1880.

——. *Organon of Homeopathic Medicine.* 2nd American ed. New York: 1843.

Hamilton, Frank Hastings. *Conversations between Drs. Warren and Putnam on the subject of medical ethics.* New York and London: 1884.

History of the Reorganization of the Boston University School of Medicine. Boston: 1918.

Hohman, Johann G. *The Long Lost Friend.* Harrisburg: 1820.

Holcombe, William. *Scientific Basis of Homeopathy.* Cincinnati: 1852.

Holmes, Oliver Wendell. *Homeopathy, and its Kindred Delusions.* Boston: 1842.

Hooker, Worthington. *Homeopathy: An Examination of its Doctrines and Evidences.* New York: 1851.

——. *Lessons from the History of Medical Delusions.* New York: 1850.

——. *Physician and Patient.* New York: 1849.

——. *The Treatment due from the Medical Profession to Physicans who become Homeopathic Practitioners.* Norwich, Connecticut: 1852.

Huston, Robert M. *An Introductory Lecture.* Philadelphia: 1846.

Leo-Wolf, William. *Remarks on the Abracadabra of the Nineteenth Century.* Philadelphia: 1835.

Letter of A. Y. P. Garnett, M.D., in reply to Henry I. Bowditch, November, 1887. Washington, D.C.: 1887.

Maclay, Edgar S. (ed.). *Journal of William Maclay.* New York: 1890.

McNaughton, James. *Annual Address before the New York State Medical Society.* Albany: 1838.

Neidhard, Charles. *An Answer to the Homeopathic Delusions of Dr. Oliver Wendell Holmes.* Philadelphia: 1842.

Okie, A. H. *Homeopathy; with Particular Reference to a Lecture by O. W. Holmes, M.D.* Boston: 1842.

Reese, David M. *The Humbugs of New York.* New York: 1838.

Roberts, John B. *Modern Medicine and Homeopathy.* Philadelphia: 1895.

Rush, Benjamin. *Medical Inquiries and Observations.* 3rd ed. Philadelphia: 1809.

Shattuck, Lemuel. *Report of the Sanitary Commission of Massachusetts, 1850.* Cambridge: 1948.

Smythe, Gonzalvo C. *Medical Heresies: Historically Considered*. Philadelphia: 1880.

Talbot, I. T. *The Common Sense of Homeopathy*. Boston: 1862.

Thacher, James. *American Modern Practice*. Boston: 1826.

Thomson, Samuel. *A Narrative of the Life and Medical Discoveries of Samuel Thomson, containing an Account of his System of Practice, and the Manner of Curing Disease with Vegetable Medicine, upon a Plan Entirely New*. 5th ed. St. Clairsville: 1829.

———. *Thomsonian Materia Medica*. 12th ed. Albany: 1841.

Trial of William Bushnell, Samuel Gregg, George Russell, David Thayer, Milton Fuller, H. L. H. Hoffendahl, I. T. Talbot, Benjamin West, all of Boston, for Practicing Homeopathy, while they were Members of the Massachusetts Medical Society. Boston: 1873.

Wesselhoeft, Robert. *Some Remarks on Dr. O. W. Holmes's Lectures on Homeopathy and its Kindred Delusions*. Boston: 1842.

Wigand, Henry. *The Principles of Homeopathic Practice as Contrasted with those of the Old School of Medicine, or Allopathy*. Boston: 1846.

Wood, George B. *A Treatise on the Practice of Medicine*. 2nd ed. Philadelphia: 1849.

F. Periodical Articles

Baker, Wyrth Post. "The Place of Homeopathy in American Medicine," *Journal of the American Institute of Homeopathy* 50 (November–December 1957): 296–98.

Bryant, Chal. "An Appeal with a Definite Program for the Establishment and Perpetuation of Homeopathic Instruction in the Universities of the United States," *Journal of the American Institute of Homeopathy* 44 (January 1951): 14–15.

Close, Stuart. "The Future of Homeopathy," *Hahnemannian Monthly* 56 (September 1921): 561–74.

———. "The Present Status of Homeopathy as Viewed by an Associate Editor of the J.A.M.A.," *Homeopathic Recorder* 39 (September 1924): 409–17; (October 1924): 459–66.

Coleman, Daniel E. S. "The Follies of Doctor Fishbein," *Journal of the American Institute of Homeopathy* 19 (February 1926): 110–21.

Devenport, C. A. "Consultation and Affiliation with Homeopathy," *Michigan Medical News* 4 (December 24, 1881): 374–75.

"Difference between Doctors," *Harper's Weekly Magazine* 37 (November 11, 1893): 1086.

Earle, Charles W. "Homeopathy as it was and how it is," *Chicago Medical Examiner* 12 (September 1871): 531–33.

Enstam, Carl. "Post-Graduate Homeopathic Education on the Pacific Coast," *Journal of the American Institute of Homeopathy* 40 (May 1947): 167–68.

Fishbein, Morris. "The Rise and Fall of Homeopathy," *American Mercury* 2 (June 1924): 150–54.

Franklin, E. C. "Homeopathy in the Army," *North American Journal of Homeopathy* 12 (November 1863): 267–78.

Henry, John H. "Is Hahnemann the Alpha and Omega of Homeopathy?" *North American Journal of Homeopathy* 10 (November 1861): 245–49.

Herzog, Lucy Stone. "A Resume of the Special Session of the House of Delegates at Chicago," *Journal of the American Institute of Homeopathy* 31 (December 1938): 736–41.

Hooker, Worthington. "The Present Mental Attitude and Tendencies of the Medical Profession," *New Englander* 10 (November 1852): 548–68.

Jackson, Edward. "Against Sectarianism in Medicine," *Medical News* 55 (October 19, 1889): 425–27.

McGraw, Theodore A. "Treatment of Inflammatory Diseases of Children by Bleeding," *Detroit Review of Medicine and Pharmacy* 1 (November 1866): 337–42.

Moore, Marcia, and Stephenson, James. "A Motivational and Sociological Analysis of Homeopathic Physicians in the U.S.A. and U.K.," *British Homeopathic Journal* 51 (October 1962): 297–303.

Morgan, W. L. "The Disintegration of the Homeopathic Profession," *Homeopathic Recorder* 24 (August 15, 1909): 339–43.

Palmer, A. B. "The Fallacies of Homeopathy," *North American Review* 134 (March 1882): 293–314.

Parker, W. W. "Was Hahnemann Insane?" *Journal of the American Medical Association* 26 (January 4, 1896): 7–9.

Parsons, James R. "Preliminary Education, Professional Training, and Practice in New York," *Journal of the American Medical Association* 26 (June 13, 1896): 1149–52.

Peterson, J. C. "On the Dissension between the Schools," *North American Journal of Homeopathy* 9 (November 1860): 308–12.

Piffard, Henry G. "The Status of the Medical Profession in the State of New York," *New York Medical Journal* 37 (April 14, 1883): 400–3.

Quine, William E. "The Medical Profession," *Journal of the American Medical Association* 32 (April 29, 1899): 980.

Rauch, John H. "Address in State Medicine," *Journal of the American Medical Association* 6 (June 12, 1886): 645–52.

Roberts, John B. "The Present Attitude of Physicians and Modern Medicine Towards Homeopathy," *Journal of the American Medical Association* 26 (February 15, 1896): 299–307.

Solis-Cohen, Solomon. "An Ethical Question," *Medical News* 55 (October 19, 1889): 427–35.

Temple, John T. "Humanity, Homeopathy and the War," *North American Journal of Homeopathy* 11 (November 1862): 161–68.

Wood, H. C. "The Medical Profession, the Medical Sects, and the Law," *New Englander* 51 (August 1889): 118–34.

Young, William W. "The Perpetuation and Propagation Program," *Journal of the American Institute of Homeopathy* 60 (July–August 1967): 198–206.

II. Secondary Sources

A. *Books*

Ameke, Wilhelm. *History of Homeopathy: Its Origins: Its Conflicts.* Edited by R. E. Dudgeon. London: 1885.

Anderson, Fannie. *Doctors Under Three Flags.* Detroit: 1951.

Bonner, Thomas N. *The Kansas Doctor.* Lawrence, Kansas: 1959.

Bradford, Thomas L. *Life and Letters of Dr. Samuel Hahnemann.* Philadelphia: 1895.

————. *The Pioneers of Homeopathy.* Philadelphia: 1897.

Burrage, Walter L. *History of the Massachusetts Medical Society.* Norwood, Massachusetts: 1923.

Burrow, James. *AMA: Voice of American Medicine.* Baltimore: 1963.

Busey, Samuel C. *Personal Reminiscences and Recollections of Forty-Six Years' Membership in the Medical Society of the District of Columbia.* Washington, D.C.: 1895.

Chicago Medical Society. *History of Medicine and Surgery and Physicians and Surgeons of Chicago, 1803–1922.* Chicago: 1922.

Cowen, David L. *Medicine and Health in New Jersey: A History.* Princeton: 1964.

Duffy, John. *History of Public Health of New York City.* New York: 1968.

————. *Rudolph Matas History of Medicine in Louisiana.* Baton Rouge: 1958–1962.

Fishbein, Morris. *A History of the American Medical Association.* Philadelphia and London: 1947.

Goodman, Nathan. *Benjamin Rush: Physician and Citizen.* Philadelphia: 1934.

Hanawalt, Leslie L. *A Place of Light: History of Wayne State University.* Detroit: 1968.

Hinsdale, Burke A. *History of the University of Michigan.* Ann Arbor: 1906.

Kelly, Howard A. *Cyclopedia of American Medical Biography.* Philadelphia and London: 1912.

Kett, Joseph F. *The Formation of the American Medical Profession.* New Haven: 1968.

King, Lester. *Medical World of the Eighteenth Century.* Chicago: 1958.

King, William Harvey. *History of Homeopathy and its Institutions in America.* New York: 1905.

Kirby, Stephen R. *The Introduction and Progress of Homeopathy in the United States.* New York: 1864.

Konold, Donald E. *History of American Medical Ethics, 1847–1912.* Madison, Wisconsin: 1962.

Massachusetts Medical Society. *A Catalogue of Its Officers, Fellows and Licentiates, 1781–1893.* Boston: 1894.

Nichols, John B., Mallory, W. J., and Wall, J. S. *History of the Medical Society of the District of Columbia, 1833–1944.* Washington, D.C.: 1947.

Norwood, William F. *History of Medical Education in the United States Before the Civil War.* Philadelphia: 1944.

Pickard, Madge E., and Buley, R. Carlyle. *The Midwest Pioneer: His Ills, Cures, and Doctors.* Crawfordsville, Indiana: 1945.

Pierce, Bessie L. *A History of Chicago.* New York: 1940.

Rosenberg, Charles E. *The Cholera Years.* Chicago: 1962.

Shryock, Richard H. *Medicine and Society in America: 1660–1860.* New York: 1960.

———. *Medicine in America: Historical Essays.* Baltimore: 1966.

———. *Medical Licensing in America, 1650–1965.* Baltimore: 1967.

Van Hoosen, Bertha. *Petticoat Surgeon.* Chicago: 1947.

Van Ingen, Philip. *The New York Academy of Medicine: Its First Hundred Years.* New York: 1949.

Waite, Frederick C. *History of the New England Female Medical College, 1848–1874.* Boston: 1950.

Walsh, James J. *History of the Medical Society of the State of New York.* New York: 1907.

Wilder, Alexander. *History of Medicine.* New Sharon, Maine: 1901.

Young, James Harvey. *The Toadstool Millionaires.* Princeton: 1961.

B. *Periodical Articles*

Berman, Alex. "The Thomsonian Movement and its Relation to American Pharmacy and Medicine," *Bulletin of the History of Medicine* 25 (September–October 1951): 405–28; (November–December 1951): 519–38.

Brieger, Gert. H. "Therapeutic Conflicts and the American Medical Profession in the 1860's," *Bulletin of the History of Medicine* 41 (May–June 1967): 215–22.

Bryan, Charles S. "Bloodletting in American Medicine, 1830–1892," *Bulletin of the History of Medicine* 38 (November–December 1964): 516–29.

Carrigan, Jo Ann. "Early Nineteenth Century Folk Remedies," *Louisiana Folklore Miscellany* 1 (January 1960): 43–64.

Duffy, John. "The Changing Image of the American Physician," *Journal of the American Medical Association* 200 (April 3, 1967): 30–34.

Jordan, Philip D. "The Secret Six: An Inquiry into the Basic Materia Medica of the Thomsonian System of Botanic Medicine," *Ohio State Archaeological and Historical Quarterly* 52 (October–December 1943): 347–55.

Kaufman, Martin. "American Medical Diploma Mills," *Bulletin of the Tulane Medical Faculty* 26 (February 1967): 53–57.

King, Lester. "The Blood-letting Controversy: A Study in the Scientific Method," *Bulletin of the History of Medicine* 35 (January–February 1961): 1–13.

Quen, Jacques M. "Elisha Perkins, Physician, Nostrum-Vender, or Charlatan," *Bulletin of the History of Medicine* 37 (March–April 1963): 159–66.

Shryock, Richard H. "Public Relations of the Medical Profession in Great Britain and the United States: 1600–1870," *Annals of Medical History*, n.s., 2 (May 1930): 308–39.

Waring, Joseph I. "The Influence of Benjamin Rush on the Practice of Bleeding in South Carolina," *Bulletin of the History of Medicine* 35 (May–June 1961): 230–37.

Young, James Harvey. "American Medical Quackery in the Age of the Common Man," *Mississippi Valley Historical Review* 47 (March 1961): 579–93.

C. *Unpublished Material*

Adams, George W. "Health and Medicine in the Union Army, 1861–1865." Ph.D. dissertation, Harvard University, 1946.

Coulter, Harris L. "Medicine and Public Opinion in the 19th Century United States." Ph.D. dissertation, Columbia University, 1969.

INDEX

Baker, Wyrth Post, 181
Barker, Fordyce, 132, 135
Barnes, Surgeon-General Joseph K., 86–87, 152–53
Barrows, Ira, 57
Bartlett, Edward G., 76
Bartlett, John S., 84
Barton, Edward H., 14
Bayard, E., 34n
Beck, John B., 5
Belais, Diana, 163
Bellevue Hospital, homeopathy in, 65–67
Bellows, Albert J., 67
Benton (folk practitioner), 17
Berkeley's Tar Water, homeopathy related to, 35–37
Bigelow, Jacob, 5
Billings, Frank, 154
Billings, Surgeon-General John S., 136
Blachford, Thomas, 33
Bliss, D. W., 73, 88–91
Blistering, 4
Blumenthal, Charles E., 116–17
Boston City Hospital, homeopathy accepted in, 151–52; homeopathy refused permission to use, 67–68
Boston Medical and Surgical Journal, description of homeopathic converts in, 33–34; expulsion of homeopaths opposed by, 78; review of Okie's pamphlet in, 43
Boston Society for the Diffusion of Useful Knowledge, 35
Boston University School of Medicine, founded, 82; homeopathy abandoned by, 171–73; permission to use Boston City Hospital given to students of, 151–52
Bowditch, Henry Ingersoll, expulsion from International Congress; fight for new code by, 135–40; paper on venesection by, 112–13
Bowditch, Nathaniel, 112
Bradford, Thomas L., 24n, 28n
Brashears, John P., 11
Brodie, William, 106
Brown, James A., 105
Browne, William F., 116
Bryan, Charles S., 110

Bryant, Chal, attempt of, to teach homeopathy at state medical schools, 181–82
Bryant, William Cullen, 34n
Buchan, William, 15–16, 21
Buchanan, John, 142
Bull, A. T., 72–73
Bull, Charles M., 12
Burrett, Claude A., 178
Burrill, General I. S., 73
Burrows, Sir George, 125
Bushnell, William, trial of, 79–85

Cabot, Richard C., 157–58
California, University of, Medical School (San Francisco), 170–71
Calomel. *See* heroic medicine
Carmichael, Thomas, 164
Carnegie Foundation, 170
Carr, C. S., 163
Cashman, W. F., 132
Cathartics. *See* heroic medicine
Chase, H. L., 85
Chicago, homeopathy in, 63–65, 175
Chicago City Hospital, dispute between homeopaths and allopaths over, 63–65
Chicago Medical Society, discussion on blood-letting in, 111; expulsion of homeopath by, 60; homeopaths in hospital opposed by, 64; organization of, 59–60
Chiropractic, 142, 161, 182
Cholera, homeopathic treatment of, 29, 93; orthodox treatment of, 12
Christian, E. P., 97
Christian Science, 142, 146, 161–62
Cinchona, Hahnemann's experimentation with, 25
Civil War, homeopathy in, 68–72, 136
Claflin, Governor (Mass.), 73–74
Clapp, Herbert C., 85, 143
Clapp, Rev. Theodore, 10
Cleveland–Pulte Medical College, 170
Close, Stuart, 173, 176–77
Colby, Isaac, 57
Cole, Hills, 164
Coleman, Daniel E. S., 177
Colfax, Vice President Schuyler, 89

postgraduate schools for, 174–75; recognition of quality of, 146, 148
Homeopathic Recorder, 169, 176–78, 181
Homeopathic statistics, 39–40
Homeopathy, American, 28–29; attacks on, 30–41, 44–46; attempts to gain specialty status for, 179–81; attitudes of, to Owen Bill, 162–66; changing allopathic attitude toward, 122–24, 126–40; changing practices of, 113–22; in Chicago, 175; debates with in organized, 148–50; defense of, 41–43, 46; development of, 23–24; elimination of, from allopathic society, 56–58, 77–86; licensure and, 144–46; in Massachusetts, 77–86; in Michigan, 93–109 passim; new code and, 139–40; in New York, 28–29, 115–17, 119–20; organization of, 55–56; rights of, in hospitals and military, 63–75; statistics on, 151; in Vermont, 183. *See also* Hahnemann, Samuel C.
Hooker, Worthington, 33; attack on homeopathy by, 44–46; evaluation of medical profession by, 50–51, 56; report on treatment due homeopaths by, 58–59
Hooper, Joseph, 113
Hoppin, Courtland, 72–73
Hospital de la Pitié (Paris), 40, 66–67
Hospitals, homeopathy in, 63–68, 146, 148–52
Hough, Joe, 182
Howe, Dr. (opposed to Thomson's practice), 20
Hubbard, Elizabeth Wright, 180
Hunt, David, 140
Huron Road Hospital (Cleveland), 175
Huston, Robert M., 33n, 52
Hutchison Sisters, song about calomel by, 13

Illinois Homeopathic Medical Association, 120–21, 160–61
Infinitesimals, Law of, development

of, 26; Hahnemannian defense of, 121–22; Holmes's ridicule of, 37–38; homeopathic embarrassment at, 114–16; homeopathic repudiation of, 114–20; Hooker's ridicule of, 44–45
Inquisition, attacks on homeopathy likened to the, 37
International Hahnemannian Association, 121–22, 181
International Medical Congress, 134–36

Jackson, Edward, 123
Jackson, J. B. S., 57
Jackson, Samuel, 5
Jacksonian democracy, 21–23, 48. *See also* Medical profession; Medical education
Jacobi, Abraham, 135, 158
Jefferson Medical College, 52
Jenner, Edward, 37
Jenner, Sir William, 125
Jesuit's Bark. *See* Cinchona
Johns Hopkins University School of Medicine, 136, 154, 171
Johnson, Gerald K., 105
Journal of the American Institute of Homeopathy, 169, 181
Journal of the American Medical Association, 147, 155, 158–59, 176

Kahlke, Charles E., 160–61
Kett, Joseph, 23
Kidd, Joseph, 125–26
King, William Harvey, 28n
"King's Evil," homeopathy kindred to the, 35–37
Kirby, Stephen R., 28n
Kittredge, Floyd G., 85–86

Leonard, C. H., 105
Leo-Wolf, Leo, attack on homeopathy by, 33
Licensure. *See* Medical licensure
Lillienthal, Professor (New Jersey homeopath), 117
Lincoln, President Abraham, 70, 86
Lippe, Adolph, statement on homeopathy by, 118–19

Lodge, E. A., 98
Louis, Pierre (Paris physician), 40
Louisiana, medical practice in, 10–12, 23
Lovett, Ezra (patient of Samuel Thomson), 20

McCall, John, 51
McCormack, J. N., 157–58
McCormack Institute, 158
McDonald, W. O., 116
McGin, J. E., 60
McGraw, Theodore A., 111
McKinley, President William, 153
McLean, Donald, 104–7
McNaughton, James, paper on homeopathy by, 32
McVickar, Brock, 63–64
Maclay, Senator William, medical treatment of, 7
March, Alden, 51
Marcy, E. E., defense of homeopathy by, 34–35
Martin, Henry A., 91
Maryland State Homeopathic Medical Society, 159
Mason, Emily, medical treatment of, 12
Massachusetts General Hospital, 82
Massachusetts Homeopathic Medical Society, 70–73, 83
Massachusetts Medical Society, dispute between A.M.A. and, 77–79; ethics violations in the, 140; expulsion of homeopaths by, 56–58, 77–86; homeopaths accepted in, 148; licensure and the, 143–44
Materia Medica Pura, written by Hahnemann, 27
Medical College of Georgia, 51
Medical education, apprenticeship in, 17–18; decline of blood-letting in, 111; decline of homeopathic, 169–77; diploma mills in American, 141–42; Flexner report on American, 168–69; in Jacksonian period, 49; low quality of, 166–67; in Michigan, 93–109; progressive reforms of, 156, 167–69; reform of, 51–52, 54–56; teaching of blood-

letting in, 2–6, 112; in West and South, 130. See also Homeopathic education
Medical ethics, code of, A.M.A. develops, 52–53; consultation clause of, 53–54; enforcement of consultation clause of, 56–62, 76–92, 105–9; the new, 125–40; revised A.M.A., 153–55
Medical licensure, 22–23, 48–50, 141–46, 160–62, 167–68; in Massachusetts, 142–44; in New Jersey, 161; in New York, 22–23, 144–46, 161–62
Medical practice, abandonment of heroic, 110–13; during age of heroic, 1–11, 15, 49–50, 122, 137; in Army, 72. See also Homeopathy, changing practice of
Medical profession, in colonial period, 15–16, 22; in Jacksonian period, 48–50; licensing of the, 141–46; reform of the, 50–62. See also Medical licensure
Michigan, University of, 93–109, 149–50, 172; threat of homeopathy at, 93–109 passim; threat of merger of two divisions of the, 149–50
Michigan State Medical Society, competition between colleges discussed in convention of, 105–6; homeopathy at the University debated in convention of, 97; lengthy debate in convention of, 103–6; orthodox practice described in a paper read before the, 111–12; resolution on homeopathy at Ann Arbor debated in convention of, 101
Middleton, Peter, 18
Military, homeopathy in, 68–74, 152–53
Miller, C. W., 163
Minnesota, homeopathic department of the University of, abandoned, 170
Minor, John C., 116–17
Minor, W. W., 60
Minot, Francis, 135

THE JOHNS HOPKINS PRESS

Designed by the Johns Hopkins Press Staff

Composed in Garamond text and display
by Monotype Composition, Inc.

Printed on 55-lb. Lockhaven
by Universal Lithographers, Inc.

Bound in Hollaston Roxite A-49234
by L. H. Jenkins, Inc.